About the Author

A finance professional who gladly quit her corporate life to don the role of wife, traveler, teacher, cook, manager, mum, writer, painter, care giver – Sohini has experienced them all.

She worked in Tata Finance Limited, a non-banking finance company in Mumbai, before moving to Kuala Lumpur due to her husband's job. She switched to marketing there and when the couple moved to Lusaka, Zambia she donned the chef's hat to cook for the entire team from the husband's office. She taught English in Accra – Ghana, contributed articles to Tokyo Timeout while living in Japan and partnered with her sister to make books more accessible to the city of Kolkata, India where together they opened a community library.

While in Melbourne, Australia she embraced ghost writing and, now a resident of California, she is still doing all the above except ghost writing – now she is writing as herself.

Dedication

To Varun, for laughing at all my jokes – poor as well as fun,
For giving my days a great start with the best coffee and the finest froth,
For making end of day special with a full bodied red,
For completing every off tune song I sing…and providing the background music,
For never giving up on me, since I was 17 ... and you 18.

To Lavanya, for rolling your eyes at my chatter,
For giving the word conscientious a deeper meaning,
For taking endurance to new heights,
For that sense of humor against all odds.

To Ditto, for your extraordinary perception, effortless compassion and unique insights.
For the simplicity and the innocence of your love,
For the goodness of your heart and kindness of your soul.

To my friends and family, for setting unsurpassable examples of beauty of human being with their kindness, goodness and excellence.
For creating, imbibing, nurturing lifelong relationships.
For making me feel blessed, every day.

To Urmila Dasgupta of Purple Folio, I will be ever grateful to you for believing that there was a story in my blog and guiding me in the right direction to make it into a book.

I doff my hat to Shilpi Banerjee for meticulously going through the manuscript. In addition to all her excellent advice_, to her I owe a great big thanks as without her scrutiny every lumbar puncture would have read as lumber puncture! Spell check can sure cause catastrophic effects.

To the reader – Thank you for reading yet another book on cancer. Just like the disease, every story is unique.

To my Publishing team – Thank you for believing in an unknown mum telling her family's story, with no publishing background, twitter presence or blog following. I stay grateful.

Sohini Rajpal

With Love from God

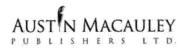

AUSTIN MACAULEY
PUBLISHERS LTD.

A CIP catalogue record for this title is available from the British Library.

ISBN 9781786293534 (Paperback)
ISBN 9781786293541 (Hardback)
ISBN 9781786293558 (E-Book)

www.austinmacauley.com

First Published (2017)
Austin Macauley Publishers Ltd.
25 Canada Square
Canary Wharf
London
E14 5LQ

Prologue

"When you come to the end of your rope,
tie a knot and hang on."

Franklin D. Roosevelt

The latte in my hand grew cold as I blindly stared at the big black screen with green blinking lights against the abbreviated names of patients in various stages of surgery. It occurred to me that I was unknowingly holding my breath oblivious to my surroundings of probably similarly disposed people – all parents, awaiting news on the surgery of their children. I felt a shiver go through me as I thought of that quiet, tired, huddled bundle on the bed that was wheeled away from me while I stood watching the doors of the OR (Operating Room) close.

I saw the light under 'pre-op' turn green against the number given to me followed by 'LAVA RAJ,' our 15-

year-old daughter's name – Lavanya Rajpal. Another parent across the room nodded, giving me a wan smile and I nodded back with probably a weak one of my own. I took a sip of my now cool latte and found that the green light I was following had moved from 'pre op' to 'in surgery.' I felt like I was in an airport terminal watching the big black board showing flight details with the name of airline, flight number, check in, security, arrival and departure. I usually picked my husband, Varun, from his work trips, sometimes waiting, sipping the latte in my hand, immersed in my kindle. But at this terminal waiting for our daughter to come out of surgery, both the kindle and latte lay untouched and neglected in my fidgeting hands. Little more than an hour later, the green light blinked at recovery and I made that much-awaited walk to see our girl, Lavanya.

I sat by her bedside waiting for the anesthesia to wear off and reflected on the month preceding the surgery. I don't know why, probably human nature, but my mind went back a month when I was looking at my child struggling with homework, an unusual sight I must add. I felt something was amiss. It is said that a mother always knows and I can truly vouch for that now. Shall I say that I felt it in my bones? Or did I feel it when I looked into her listless eyes and drooping shoulders or did the thought occur to me when I heard her say, "Hey mommy, you want to sit with me while I complete homework?"

To rule out a recurrence of the disease, which practically snatched her childhood away when she was five years old, I made an appointment with her pediatrician. We noticed small red dots on her calves the next day and I blessed Google as I discovered that they could be something called petechia, a condition caused by possible low platelets, a component of blood responsible for preventing bleeding. Call me silly but I phoned the doctor and tried to reschedule the appointment to the earliest possible day. The next day, barely twelve hours later, I received a picture that Lavanya had clicked of her arm at lunchtime in school with a message that said, "Hey mommy, the dots are on my arms now."

The red dots had appeared on her arms around noon and by the time I picked her up after a couple of hours, her mouth was full of black king-sized blisters. I headed directly to the doctor's clinic not waiting for the scheduled appointment two days hence and the very kind doctor took us in just because I, the mother, had a bad feeling or an inkling. Lavanya looked healthy enough except for her complaint of, "Hey mommy, I am so tired!" Blood works were done and we were sent home with the instruction to await the doctor's call in three to four days with the results.

With labs done after school around 5.00 p.m., the call came in less than 15 hours, with my phone ringing just after our 11-year-old son Ditto left for school the following morning. I recall the date, the time, even where I was sitting and exactly what I was doing when I heard that devastating news on the phone from a very matter of fact doctor, who advised me to head to Stanford Children's Hospital's ER (Emergency Room) at the earliest. He had kindly called them ahead and we were expected.

I remember the internal shivers I had and, on reminiscing, I now know what is meant by 'heart dropped to my stomach' or 'couldn't breathe.' There was a strange

11

kind of empty feeling, a hollowness which seemed to conquer my body and mind.

The diagnosis of blood cancer, leukemia again, at 15 years of age after being in remission for 10 years seemed to be squeezing my heart, lungs, intestines and everything that was within me. I sightlessly brought out my diary and began making a quick list of things I needed to do before I drove to the hospital, all the time trying my husband's phone who was on a work trip in Mumbai, India. The top of the list said 'find address of Stanford Children's Hospital,' followed by, 'call Ditto's school and arrange for him to be with someone.'

So it happened that on Marc 26th 2013, at 8.05 a.m. to be precise, I left my morning cuppa half way through to wake our tired daughter in order to head to the hospital. For a girl who had been there and done that when she was five years old I was surprised to hear, "I hope I can be back in time to appear for my chemistry test tomorrow!" This was a diagnosis made in her sophomore year, in grade ten, as a 15-year-old, that changed her life completely. At times it dragged her a few steps back but her will power, courage and zest for life pushed her far ahead than behind. One step behind and two-steps forward was what I would aptly call the long tedious journey. I thought I must share her story that I had been told by many people had inspired them, touched them and pushed them beyond the expected.

Chapter 1

When one lives in eight countries in twenty years, one gains not one or two but multiple families and friends of different races, religions and nationalities. When home is not limited to one city, but comprises of many small towns and big cities, one gets introduced to an array of people, social customs, norms, foods, festivals, languages, laws, music and much more, developing a love for many things foreign and respecting several others. Varun and I have been married for over two decades and in those we have moved ten times, having lived in India – our home country, Malaysia, Japan, Zambia, Ghana, Jamaica, Australia and now America. He is a north Indian and yours truly is from Bengal in the east. Our wedding ceremony was not limited to a combination of ceremonies and rituals from both our communities but also encompassed communities our family members were married into.

It was an interesting, fun and educational wedding ceremony if I may say so now! Our wedding fineries and jewelries included something from different parts of the country depending on where an aunt was based or from which state the uncle originated. We did look kind of funny, slightly strange, but the happiness of marrying each other overshadowed the strange multi-cultural outfits and we didn't complain. We were aware that Indian weddings were nothing about the bride or the groom but all about their families, neighbors and the entire community.

We began our married life by moving into a one-bedroom apartment provided by Varun's company. We proudly drove to our new home barely, 650 square feet in area, in a borrowed car with all our worldly possessions fitted into a few suitcases.

Mumbai, where every square foot is very precious and extremely expensive, how thrilled were we to find that our new home had not one but two bathrooms! We were spoilt with that luxury. The living room and bedroom overlooked the beautiful mountains part green, part brown, dotted with slums having a million habitations, no way a deterrent to our enthusiasm! I realized that where there is love, there is only happiness.

Mumbai life entailed early morning rise and shine, auto rickshaw ride to the station, train to the CBD (Central Business District), walk or cab to work and the same reversed in the evening. For those who haven't been introduced to an auto rickshaw yet, I must explain that it's a three-wheeler contraption meant for three passengers, an Indian invention for those short commutes that the regular cab won't do. The driver of the vehicle perched precariously on a little rectangle platform like seat in the front while the three passengers squeezed onto a longer similar platform like seat at the back hanging on for dear life while the driver did an Indiana Jones on Mumbai lanes. It's another story altogether that the further one went from the city into the suburbs, those same vehicles designed for three passengers accommodated often close to six, all hanging onto each other for dear life. The beauty of it all is that no one got off in a bad temper or foul mood. In fact one might just spot those alighted waving a rare mix of fond and exasperated goodbyes to the departing vehicle. It was just the Mumbai way of life.

When the transfer to Kuala Lumpur came soon after, the same enthusiasm took us readily and happily to the new country, our first foreign travel. Both our parents had been world travelers. My sister was married to a Captain in the Merchant Navy and she too, was world travelled. So, when it was us flying overseas, we had the best wishes of both our families with a long list of dos and don'ts. After all, we were just 25 and 26 years old respectively. We were considered naïve, simple, innocent, foolish, gullible and much more, but let's avoid unnecessary details.

By the time our first-born Lavanya made an appearance, we had been married for three years, having lived in Malaysia, India and Zambia. We had agonizing fourteen hours of labor followed by C-section to bring our girl into this beautiful world. The husband, a north Indian having scant knowledge of Bengali, was left confused when my Bengali family and friends wearing big smiles repeated over and over on the telephone and to those present, "May Hoeche, May Hoeche." Literally translated, it was a tad confusing as it meant May had happened and we were in the middle of October. But 'May' in Bengali means 'girl' so simplified it meant a girl had happened or announced the birth of a girl.

Despite being one of the first countries to have a woman as the Prime Minister as well as the President of the nation, India is a huge contradiction. The birth of a girl could either trigger celebrations similar to the birth of a boy, or it could also bring a pall of gloom. We fell in the former group and the birth of Lavanya left us in a constant state of glee, an inexplicable, indescribable happiness because she was a gift of our love. I find discussions on family planning strangely ironical, because very honestly, we cannot plan a baby. We simply can't plan miracles of life just because they are gifts from God.

She was all of three months of age when I packed her into her basinet and travelled to Kingston, Jamaica via London Heathrow and Gatwick from Mumbai to join Varun, who was on an assignment there. After 20 hours of flying, four hours of transit with a long bus ride between the two airports in London, I was convinced that I was mad to have attempted the journey with a few months old baby without the husband. Over and above that, both sets of our parents were not familiar to the baby being carried in the basinet, as to them it was just a piece of luggage and not a safe baby carrier. What if Sohini left it behind with the baby! Imagine forgetting your basinet, baby included, at airport check-in! Now I realize why in India elders believe that girls should be married at a tender young age. Had I been older, I would have been (hopefully) wiser and I would have never contemplated on attempting this foolhardy journey, and that too, all by myself. I must admit at this juncture there have been differences in opinion about me being wise (er) with age, but I will skip those musings. Varun still laughs as he regales us with stories of the mother-daughter sleep cycle in the week of arrival in Jamaica. He didn't see us awake when he returned from work every evening nor were we up when he left in the mornings! Not that he complained. He liked how he looked. Sleep deprived new mums are known to have landed their fists on the poor husbands.

To cut a long story short, our girl had her first birthday in Ghana; second in Jamaica; third in Japan; fourth in India and by then her little brother had arrived. This was the year 2001 and the birth of our boy was shared with the world by way of text messages from tiny Nokia phones and mails from Dell laptops. Had it been 2015, probably there would have been instant messages in addition to selfies all over FB, Instagram and tweets of the new update from iPhone.

I recall Lavanya's admission test to kindergarten as though it happened yesterday. I must add that the husband shudders at my 'exceptionally' humble ability to remember incidents. The principal had asked her the father's name. Promptly and very smartly had come the reply, Varun Rajpal. To the query of honey what is your mother's name, equally smartly followed the answer, Sohini Aunty. In India all women who happen to be the parents' friends are called aunty and all the men are uncle. Since all her friends called me Sohini aunty our girl thought that's what my name was. Simple! Just like with the parents being big fans of musicians like Sting, Pink Floyd, both our children since childhood have watched a few Sting and Roger Water/Pink Floyd concerts and very simply would discuss the music of Sting uncle and Pink Floyd uncle! And yes, we do like Deep Purple uncle too and appreciate Reo uncle. Now reminiscing, I wonder why they never got around to saying Madonna aunty. She stayed the universal Madonna!

Lavanya was the perfect little lady, eager to learn, with a strong mind and loving heart. I recalled her excitement about going to school and her horror on realizing mum didn't stay back, learning to join dots, color, make standing lines, sleeping lines, slanting lines and graduating to writing alphabets.

The move to Tokyo, new school, new friends and the adjustments at a tender age of three was taken in her stride. Her school was on a busy street and every morning volunteers would stand on either side of the blind turn calling out, "Car is coming, car is coming!" to help kids and parents navigate the blind corner. So much so, that at any blind corner thereafter, car or no car, our girl would exaggeratedly peep around the corner and mime exactly like the volunteers innocently calling, "Car is coming, car is coming." Yes, she thought, that's what one said when one stood by or passed a blind corner.

We call our boy Ditto simply because he is a ditto copy of his dad. He turned out to be a one in a million baby with his cheery disposition and happy personality. Raised in Tokyo he was the only one-year-old I know who bowed deep on meeting people and bowed deep again on parting. He inculcated the Japanese way of life just by observing;

no one had to tell him about respect, it just grew on him naturally. Observation and experience are said to be the greatest teachers and time and again he proved it right because another Japanese custom he picked up was the art of saying or waving goodbye. After that deep bow, he would wave his little hands rapidly until the person he was bidding adieu to, was out of sight. It was common in Tokyo to see schoolgirls waving bye to their friends standing outside stations for an extended time. So I couldn't really blame him as I crossed the always busy Shibuya station very often pushing his stroller.

He hero-worshipped his older sister, though over the years that one aspect has changed. I realize that siblings and hero-worshipping do not really gel together. They love each other but expressing that would be rare, the healthy fights and arguments are more expressions of love than hugs and kisses. He followed her around then and imitated things she did. He does follow her around now, but only for help in say, math or advice on essay. I loved spending time with our children. I got to hear and feel their simplicity and love. For example, our little boy on a very energetic day would hold my face and exclaim, "A hundred kisses," and kiss me a hundred times, counting till hundred at a breakneck speed, while our girl would smile primly and give a very precise kiss on the cheek with the right pressure for exactly the right amount of time. Joys of motherhood kept multiplying as days became years.

Chapter 2

*"One laugh of a child will make
the holiest day more sacred still."*

Robert G Ingersoll

Ditto was just over a year old when his hero-worshipped, lovely, serene and calm sister was diagnosed with the dreaded disease, cancer of the blood – leukemia at a tender age of five. Who would have thought that the simple stomach and hip aches that began in Tokyo were also one of the symptoms of blood cancer? Who could have imagined that the disease would escape diagnosis because nothing wrong appeared in repeated labs, ultra sounds, CT scans, X-rays and extensive blood draws done in Tokyo? To put it mildly we were devastated, though greatly relieved too, because we finally had a diagnosis of the infrequent but mysterious pain. I had thought that these things were limited to movies and fiction novels. That it could be non-fiction and this close to home was unimaginable. That a simple stomach and hip ache could be cancer was a revelation. That a child who looked healthy, jumped around playfully, twirled on her toes to imaginary music, giggled happily, ate and drank healthily was in fact walking around with her WBC falling to unbelievable low levels, platelets dangerously low and an immune system weak with the disease that stayed unknown until my 34th birthday, seemed to be the worst nightmare ever. I aged overnight on my birthday and Varun just a year older than me at 35 cried hysterically as he broke the news to me. This was India, the doctor didn't break the news of cancer to the mother, you see!

After the initial shock, tears and fears, we pulled ourselves together to wage war against the disease, growing older, matured and much more responsible than I could ever have imagined us to be in a matter of days. With the birth of a baby, one does become responsible or tries to be. But when the baby is diagnosed with a disease like cancer, the magnitude of the responsibility grows exponentially. We saw ourselves promising to lead a happy and healthy life maintaining as much normalcy as possible in our lives, while the traumatizing treatment began. We didn't indulge in any movie style talks or discussions with God, we didn't yell, we didn't fight or even ask or wonder why her! Why us? It had happened and we were determined to see her and us through it. She was in grade one, just back to Mumbai from Tokyo and she taught us lessons on patience and perseverance.

I can't imagine a five-year-old cooped indoors day after day, month after month, unable to go out to play due to fear of infection. Did she complain? No, not once! With the Hickman catheter, a foreign body inserted into her by a small surgical process, all kinds of precautions were to be taken to avoid infection. The catheter helped in treatment with blood draw, administration of chemo drugs into her without multiple needle pokes. A little pipe through her jugular vein reached close to her heart, with one end popping out of her chest, this catheter was a blessing. Varun and I became adept at flushing and cleaning the catheter with saline and heparin. She had to give up going to school and I taught her at home everything that she was learn at school.

Almost in complete isolation with close to zero immunity Lavanya's life underwent a huge change. An adult can understand the reasons for that change and adjust along with it. But for a five-year-old with no understanding about the disease and reasons for isolation, just to co-operate with doctor's instructions and with parents following them, required an understanding and maturity beyond her age. She didn't protest, didn't throw a tantrum, just had one question for Varun, "Daddy what's wrong with me?" Varun explained it very simply. His explanation was that, there was a 'kida' (bug) which was making her sick. Our aim was to take the medicines that unfortunately didn't come as tablets that one could swallow easily, but as IV or IM injections to kill that kida/the bug. The Hickman catheter facilitated treatment without the pain of constant needle probes. The chemo administered brought all blood counts like WBC (white blood cells), hemoglobin, platelets to very low levels raising the risk of infection, as did the presence of a foreign body like the catheter inside her body for an extended period of time leading to isolation and it was all one big vicious circle. So, the presence of the Hickman catheter was to avoid the pain of pokes and the requirement of extra care came in because the Hickman catheter was a foreign body. The counts depleted with chemo so the necessity of isolation. Our motto became, 'kill the kida' meaning 'kill the bug.' Our boy barely able to form words would exclaim with a big toothless gummy smile, his podgy little hands thrown up in the air, "Killkalliyyya." It was a cry of victory where nothing could go wrong and the family stood united to bring about that victory with medication, isolation, prayers, positive thinking and a whole lot of gratitude for all the help we received. The clarion call of killing the bug was accompanied by another motto of keeping their childhood happy and normal despite the grave situation.

On reflection, the incidents that play before me from our first tryst with leukemia treatment is not of the harrowing painful chemotherapy or radiation but that of a six-year-old Lavanya with a beautiful shining pate, wearing a wide smile, dancing the night away with her dad, bringing in the New Year.

The highlights of those times are not the long drives to and from the hospital every day in crawling Mumbai traffic or walking the endless corridors of the hospital, but that of our friends playing outside the facility with our little boy, while Varun and I spent time together with Lavanya in her isolated room. We bought books and more books of all kinds. Indian mythology, joke books, mystery books, Enid Blytons, Nancy Drews, books on riddles and puzzles and she devoured them while taking breaks to throw up in the basin next to her. The puzzles, riddles, quizzes and jokes turned out to be contagious, as soon doctors and nurses coming to check on Lavanya would be either armed with a new riddle to ask, a puzzle to solve or sometimes the doctor would sit back to play a game of UNO or one of the multiple board games we kept in her room. At one time I stepped out of her room only to find one of the nurses doing some serious thinking while she prepared to walk in with chemo and a mother of all riddles for our girl. There was glee on the nurse's face and anticipation on Lavanya's and no one cared for the toxic drugs that were trickling into her veins.

When home, the siblings bonded over everything and nothing since they were each other's companions and best friends. She understood his vocabulary when none of us could. How could one decipher his excitement that 'boagaya' meant Bob the Builder cartoon? When she wanted to bike in the evenings with the little brother following on his tricycle, we pushed our dining table aside and *voila!* the kids could ride inside the house. Mind you, this was Mumbai, where homes are comparable to pigeonholes, small and compact, but the kids didn't complain that they had to bike in the dining room. Round and round they went as I sat reading at the table, with my head spinning from their circular motions. It was a grueling two and half years long treatment and the day dawned for the last chemo coinciding with her eighth birthday on 17th Oct 2005. With diagnosis on my birthday 29th July 2003, it was little more than two years. It was said then, that if the disease didn't relapse within five years of diagnosis, one was considered cured and the possibility of getting the disease was the same as for those who had never had it. So once year 2008 came, marking the five years since diagnosis, we breathed easy and were ready to move on, with Varun being transferred to Melbourne, Australia.

My dad worked for the Indian Government and we had moved around within India, schooling in Central Schools whereby the syllabus, books, uniforms remained the same all over the country, with changes only in the city, teachers and friends. Our children were challenged by something more as their dad worked in a company with global presence and they had the good fortune, in the eyes of many the 'misfortune' of living in four continents and gaining education in three, making their FB page look like the United Nations.

The school in Melbourne found Lavanya above her age dictated grade in academics and decided to start her in grade seven instead of the age appropriate grade six to continue to challenge her abilities and help her grow. So while she was eleven years old her classmates were going onto thirteen. There were quite a few adjustment issues. She was still into dolls, Enid Blytons and Harry Potter while her peers were into makeup, dating and Dan Brown. Our boy was in an age appropriate grade of second grade and fitted right in. In the second week of his school he received a certificate for, "Exemplary behavior and respect for peers and teachers as well as school property." Not surprising, as at two and half years of age he had received the "Most well-adjusted child in kindergarten."

Melbourne was beautiful and Varun and the kids adapted themselves to Melbourne weather of experiencing all four seasons in one day. It was not surprising to see them walking out in the mornings with umbrellas, sweating during the hot day and wearing a jacket against the cold in the evenings. We spent good four years enjoying the Aussie way of life. Our kids played all possible sports with regular academics. Lavanya rowed in the lake across the school, took a dip with the ducks when her boat capsized, returned home thrilled with herself and life, so what if there was duck poo stuck onto her straight long hair! Ditto played footie, the Aussie style football and fell in love with the game. We made some great friends, with whom I know that friendship will last a lifetime despite distances and time differences as unknown to us then, the wheels were working to get us onto our next destination across the globe.

While in Melbourne we were exposed to the best humor in the world – the Aussie sense of humor is unbeatable. It begins when the accent hits you on arrival at immigration, when the official would give a big smile to exclaim, "Welcome to Australia, and why are you here, to die (today)?" While the new entrant might just murmur, "No, no, I haven't come here to die, I have come here to work or I am a tourist," until the accent grew on them. Incidents that still send me into fits of giggles even when alone, are many. Once while walking home on St Kilda road I laughed hysterically when I spotted a bus that was not in service, but the driver was innovative with the sign on top of the bus saying – "Lost and don't care." Then there was a time I was going into CBD and the ever-punctual public transport was a few minutes late. The tram driver lightened the moment by making an announcement on the public address system for all passengers to hear, "We are running five minutes behind, due to very strong head winds!"

I loved Melbourne and realized one doesn't need to take life seriously. It happens continuously, while we probably constantly make plans for it. Very recently we had an Aussie colleague and friend visiting and Varun's relatives dropped by at the same time. Before we could make the introductions this Aussie walked out of the kitchen and in that oh so lovable Aussie drawl introduced himself, "Hi, I am the family butler," to our surprised relatives.

We attended the subject selection for grade 11 and at around the same time realized it was that time of our lives again – we were moving. Lavanya was devastated! She wasn't delighted about the move at all and wondered if she could stay back to complete year 12 in Melbourne. Ditto, too, was upset but his excitement about the move overshadowed his feelings of leaving Melbourne and all things familiar. Lavanya had been excited about the subjects she had chosen for the IB (International Baccalaureate) curriculum and was looking forward to the new school year in six months' time. How different siblings could be! I realized it was that difference in siblings despite similar genes that helped to balance a family.

While we empathized with her feelings we were not comfortable about leaving her so far away from us because our move was 16,000 plus kilometers, 10,000 plus miles away, back into the northern hemisphere. Yes, we had to learn to talk in miles from then on because we were moving to the United States of America.

Chapter 3

"We keep moving forward, opening new doors and doing new things, because we are curious and curiosity keeps leading us down new paths."

Walt Disney

So we were moving! This time from kilometers to miles, liters to gallons, 240 volts to 120 volts, right hand driving to left-hand driving, mate (maite) to dude, and the list was endless. The move to the United States from Australia was a huge one. Despite having been there and done that before, it was never to this vast a distance or such a huge change that affected all aspects of our life. We added yet another driving license to the wallet, discarded the Aussie credit cards and store cards, replacing them with their American counterparts. Myers became Macys, David Jones was equivalent of Nordstrom and Bunnings was replaced by Home Depot.

Having experienced private schooling in Melbourne, we chose a district with renowned schools and settled into a small town well known for its public schools, excellent school district and safe environment. Just some of the top check boxes one ticks when looking for a place to live and raise a family. Until we arrived in Silicon Valley we had thought that Melbourne was multi-racial, with a lovely cocktail of cultures. Silicon Valley gave the word 'multi' a completely new broader meaning. What an eclectic mix of color, race, religion and nationality, making a complete newcomer feel at home instantly and we even began spelling colour as color!

Having lived predominantly in Commonwealth nations, America was a surprise and I started counting the hit me on the face differences right away. Driving on the right side of the road and California allows a right turn on a red light unless otherwise specified! Dates changed from dd/mm/yy to mm/dd/yy. Why oh why! I couldn't begin to count how many cheques I had to cancel and then of course the cheques became checks. I learned that the small cappuccino is the tall one and that, too, should be ordered only when my better half was present to share with me and likewise for food portions. Everything was gigantic! The plates were larger, the glasses bigger, their diameters wider! Meanwhile, mates became dudes and July became summer, not winter or monsoon! I never had to stand in a queue again as they became lines, which yours truly realized only after infinite blank looks on enquiry of, "Is this where the queue begins?" One of my first purchases on moving into our new home was a footstep ladder. I couldn't reach the overhead shelves and I considered myself 'tall' standing proud at 5 ft. 4 inches. The temperature was measured in Fahrenheit, weight in pounds and height in centimeters. I was buying gas by the gallon. Petrol and 'liter' seemed long lost friends. Do note the liter and not litre! I was never proud of my math, and the amount of conversions that daily life entailed, I almost lost whatever numbers I knew. And then I would come home and to switch on the light, I actually had to turn it off! The switches worked upside down. I seriously needed divine intervention to survive. When buying a car, Ditto and I were pleased that it came with a sunroof but the salesman looked at us quizzically and remarked, "You do mean the moon roof don't you?" Now I take the liberty to claim that I am 'slightly' more knowledgeable because I discovered there is actually a difference between the two. Go google! And one common aspect worldwide is that, unknown to us Google- the noun became google- the verb.

Well, we learned and reached a comfort level soon. Why blame America! I recall when we moved to our new home in Japan I had the biggest and the most beautiful refrigerator that I had ever owned or seen. I had almost shaken with excitement while arranging the fresh vegetables, fruits, chicken and fish in their designated spots only to find the tomato frozen the next morning and the chicken looking miserable. It was an upside down fridge, unknown in the 1990s in India but very prevalent everywhere now.

At the risk of sounding cliché, life was beautiful. Despite all the changes and many embarrassing episodes, I loved America. Seven months into this honeymoon period, a demon from the past resurfaced with renewed vengeance.

Our daughter, a sophomore, was (re) diagnosed with leukemia. Our girl was struck with cancer for the second time in her 15 years of life and all she was concerned about was the chemistry test the following day.

To cut a long sordid story short, after multiple attempts over 6 hours to find a vein good enough to draw blood to confirm diagnosis, the vascular team was brought in to the ER to help set up a PICC line and an IV. Thereafter my girl was sent off to the Pediatric Intensive Care Unit with the final confirmed diagnosis of Acute Lymphoblastic Leukemia, high risk as on diagnosis her WBC was at 460000 and age was 15. The PICC line is a Peripherally Inserted Central Catheter that would facilitate treatment without multiple injections and troublesome vein hunting. Varun had already cut short his visit in Mumbai and left for home when it all began and our friend Nafis flew in from the East Coast to give us support and help until his arrival.

Since we had friends and family in four continents, the hospital was flooded with phone calls enquiring on the status of Lavanya with news traveling by word of mouth. As the hospital was inundated with calls from all over the globe, the nurses introduced us to *www.mylifeline.org*, a website especially for cancer patients to reach out to be engulfed in a circle of love and hope by giving periodic updates on patient as well as any help needed by family. The website could either be public or private as per the writer's/family's wish. They needed to post the details they wished to share with those invited to be a part of the website. So we registered our website with limited access, by invitation only to family and friends, spread from Tokyo in the east to California in the west.

What began as little updates from us turned into something much bigger, initiating discussions, debates, prayers and formation of unique friendships between people who came together as one. It wove an invisible, intangible bond amongst strangers, who connected on the blog towards a common cause of providing moral support to a teen with cancer and her family. The oldest person on it would be seventy plus years and the youngest a teenager but irrespective of their age, race, nationality, culture and background they empathized as one, all the time encouraging and supporting us through the treatment. The beauty of the website was that it was not just me sharing our day-to-day life through the treatment. It was beyond that, as family and friends poured in their thoughts, concern, love and prayers into words that made it as special as it became eventually. Much as I would love to help others in similar situations, the active treatment period does not give anyone much time or energy to talk to people, let alone go somewhere to counsel another. The website claims, 'No cancer patient should ever feel alone,' and that's exactly what happened.

We were connected to everyone despite the geographical distances. When we reached the end of the intense treatment, many of our friends felt that the story should be shared so that others in similar situation or any difficult situation knew that there was something beyond medicines, chemotherapy, side effects and sickness. They will get re-introduced to possibilities given birth by a positive state of mind, a sense of moving forward against all odds, to not just be a survivor but to prevail and accomplish, to go from strength to strength to achieve, to convert and conquer dreams into realities.

Each patient has his or her own unique story, each story very different from the other but the unique common factor amongst all was that strong conscious or sub conscious belief rooted deep within that, a day will dawn when they will be cancer free. Each family worked with a belief and the one that worked for us was that when we accepted whatever God bestowed upon us with love and gratitude, it created miracles and thereby I named our story, *"With Love from God."*

Chapter 4

"Gratitude can transform common days into thanksgiving;
turn routine jobs into joy and change ordinary
opportunities into blessings."

William Arthur Ward

When Lavanya had been diagnosed with leukemia in Mumbai, a grade one child, she was an epitome of grace, co–operating at every step. So, the treatment was a cakewalk, with some expected side effects and some unexpected hiccups. That was in the year 2003, at Lilavati Hospital, Mumbai. My engineer husband and the finance professional me, had learned about WBC, platelets, neutropenia, hemoglobin, isolation, drug toxicity among many other things. WBC, the White Blood Cells are responsible for fighting infections while platelets help in healing by preventing bleeding by forming blood clots. Hemoglobin carries oxygen from the lung to the tissues and carbon dioxide back to the lungs from them. Biology learned in high school came flooding back, only now it held a lot more meaning. My weak math had perked up with mental calculations of ANC – the Absolute Neutrophil Count, derived by multiplying the percentage of neutrophil with the WBC, on a daily basis. And just when we had thought that it was all over and behind us it was back, with vengeance this time, involving a lot more in the form of side-effects and unexpected hiccups as a teenager's reaction are known to be more volatile than a five-year old child's. Tell me about it! Of course in the ten years since, my math had become rusty again and I blessed Steve Jobs for iPhone that became an extension of my body, for her to call me when she needed me from across the house or to calculate ANC. I couldn't do that mentally any more. How quickly had the ability at mental math been delegated to a gadget!

Year 2013, California, America, Lucile Packard Children's Hospital at Stanford became a second home. Fortunately, barely 15 miles from our actual home, the travel was not as traumatic as the first time in Mumbai. Ten years on we saw her getting almost the same medications in a different regime, a more intense chemotherapy, but without the radiation that she received the first time in Mumbai.

The treatment Lavanya received was divided into phases, called induction, consolidation, interim maintenance 1, delayed intensification, interim maintenance 2 and thereafter regular maintenance lasting two years from the start of interim maintenance, with the entire treatment lasting close to two and half years. Today as I write our story, I do wonder as to who on earth gave the treatment phases those names, huh!

Some of the therapies were administered by IV infusion over a period of time, some were IV push and some were intra muscular while another was by way of lumbar puncture usually done under general anesthesia. Before heading to the procedure fasting, patients would go through the colorful enticing menu to order food they would eat when allowed after the procedure. The menu looks very interesting in the first weeks in the hospital but as the stays become more often and of longer duration, one starts overlooking it. The colorful menu lies neglected initially and forgotten eventually.

With time we realized that despite having gone through leukemia treatment before, we were new to the disease. The age of the child played a huge role in the side effects of the drugs and their toxicity. As days turned into weeks and then into months we learned a lot, gained tremendously and started reflecting an inner gratitude unknown in the circumstances. We learned of a new kind of circle, the circle of gratefulness, gratitude and appreciation. We learned that the more we were grateful and were full of gratitude, the more reasons God gave us to feel them again and again. This whole gamut of feelings was brought about by our friends who held our hand, wiped our tears, listened to our fears, encouraged our hopes, made us laugh. To put it simply, they gave themselves. They gave themselves in phone calls, writing comments on the updates that I posted on the blog, sending texts, e-mails, snail mails, presents and visits. Most importantly they gave their time in doing all above and more. There were many of them and I cannot do justice in writing about what their being with us accomplished, neither can I name each and every one of them as each one was special. I have taken the liberty of mentioning some with their kind permission.

Before we knew it the school support had kicked in. Teachers and friends made up Lavanya's stream of visitors and each one brought something funny, interesting, informative and often endearing. Her Chemistry teacher Mia Onodera came with huge posters with messages from her classmates and teachers. Each class had made a different poster with drawings, thoughts and messages. She received these from her French, Chemistry, Math and Literature class and has preserved them all for putting up in her room when she grows up and buys that big house with huge walls to cover them with messages from her high school friends when she was unwell. One message said, "Hi, I am wishing you a speedy recovery. I sit behind you in class." I realized she didn't really know the person but received messages wishing her recovery. I found one message particularly funny that said, "Hey get well soon. I am the new boy." So, the class had a new boy who had heard about this absent girl undergoing treatment and added his wishes too. It is said that children are a reflection of God and I would agree on that and further add that it's true irrespective of the age of the child or country of origin. Another message that warmed me was from a girl she barely knew in school saying, "You can do it again, just as you did before and just as I did a few months back." I realized that cancer is striking more often, but then it doesn't stand a chance against the grit and determination of those stricken.

The Math teacher Sushma Bana dropped by. The lovely Indian lady very kindly offered to do my Indian grocery shopping, as my local friends wouldn't know what to shop. Someone I had never met before, someone whose role in our lives till then was just teaching Math to our daughter, became another unexpected support as she let us know from time to time that she was going to the temple in Sunnyvale to pray for her. I admit I had not been to a temple, I had been praying at home so I felt good that there were people visiting all holy places, temple, chapel, mosque and church to offer prayers for our girl. The thoughtful Chemistry teacher sent experiments that could be safely done at home to keep Lavanya both occupied and interested. The French teacher Sarah Finck wrote her a letter in French, sending her medals home by post and became a regular visitor, while the young literature teacher Frank Ruskus brought in reinforcements in the form of another teacher, as he didn't know what he would talk to his teenage student about. Both he and the student were pleasantly surprised that they could converse happily at length. Prior to his visit she had expressed to me, "Hey mommy what would we talk about? He walks up and down the aisle between rows in class when he teaches; he never sits when he talks, he is always on the move, how will he do that here in the hospital room? Where will he walk!" The teacher was most amused on hearing her thoughts.

On one hand the hospital corridors became as familiar as the corridor between our bedrooms and on the other hand our friends around the world shrunk the distances keeping their online vigil. We kept hearing and reading about the things they did in places they considered holy for our girl's recovery, with some attempting to even bribe the God Almighty by foregoing or giving up their favorite drink or food. Rachna in Kuala Lumpur gave up her favorite cuppa until Lavanya returned home fine, Krishna from Singapore walked up the Tirupati Balaji Temple in India to have a one on one with God to help in her recovery. For this he had to fly from Singapore to Chennai, India, hire a car to reach the foothills of the temple and then walk uphill overnight. Gina my neighbor walked over and held my hand as she closed her eyes and prayed in her own way. Jayshree and Shilpi started prayer meetings and chanting in not just the city they lived in but across the world. Alka initiated Buddhist chanting with her group of friends. Some went to church, some to temples and others to mosques. Some prayed at the Fire Temple, others chanted Buddhist mantras at home alone and more often in a group. I imagined if Gods from all religions had a United Nations in heaven they would definitely find prayers for a certain teenager common amongst them. When Lubna came to help with hospital stay during the initial days both Varun and I were touched. What moved us immensely was her firm belief in her prayers, as every morning she would cover her head and sit by Lavanya's head reading the Holy Quran. My neighbor Gina read the Holy Bible and prayed to her Lord for exactly the same wish that Lubna prayed to her Prophet. Priya and Poulomi from Mumbai drove to Shirdi while Mamta sent blessings from the Gurdwara at Amritsar and Priya from Delaware prayed at her Church.

These were all people we met, became friends with, in different cities, during various stages of our lives and they have stayed with us in our hearts despite not being in the same city. Shilpi is my high school friend, yes, I have known her for more than thirty years since we were both in our blue skirt and white blouse uniform with two pigtails. Lubna and Alka are wives of Varun's colleagues and our husbands have worked together for more than two decades. All this talk of knowing them for decades does make me feel ancient. Jayshree and Krishna are friends we made in Mumbai as our children were in the same school and we lived in the same building. Mamta's and Poulomi's daughters and Lavanya have been friends for fifteen years since they were two years old. As I read this to Lavanya she said, "Hey, mommy, I too am old, I have the same friends for fifteen years!" As I think back I realize that many of our friends are spread around the world far away in different continents, hemispheres but technology along with the wish to stay connected has kept us entwined in each other's daily lives and my gratitude for that wish as well as technology is endless. I soon realized that being too busy to stay connected is a myth, finding time is solely dependent on that wish to find the time and we as a family were warmed by how much time our friends and family had for us despite their own hectic schedules.

Chapter 5

*"At Starbucks I like ordering a tall venti
in a grande cup. That's basically me asking for
a small large in a medium cup."*

Jarod Kintz

Before going for lumbar punctures Lavanya would peruse
the extensive menu and order something so that once she
woke up from anesthesia there would be food waiting for
her. It was difficult for a teenager to fast for the frequent
lumbar punctures. At one instance she ordered a baked
potato. When it arrived we did stare at it in awe and then at
each other as we smothered giggles lest we appeared rude
to the person delivering it. We have eaten baked potato in
India, Australia, Japan and Zambia among other places and
they all looked very different from the version served here.
In Tokyo for example, it had miso, wasabi, sometimes
scallion stuffed in it and looked beautiful, intricate, delicate

just as all things Japanese do. As far as presentation was concerned it was picture perfect. I would touch it gingerly with a fork to avoid ruining the beauty of the dish. In India the baked/boiled potato is roughly cut, followed by boiled garbanzo beans, chopped raw onion, roasted peanuts, green chilies and spices presented in a little bowl made with leaves. To be truthful it won't make you gasp in wonder, smelled far from delicate, the very opposite of its Japanese counterpart. But it did look interesting, made one environment conscious with the use of that bowl made with leaves, so what if it fired up your entire digestive system and you had fumes coming out of your ears. The Aussie version had rosemary, chives, sweet chilies, turmeric, you name it and they had it. They would play around with spices and herbs, slapping some, throwing others and generally having fun while doing it all, presenting one with a very casual but delicious version of baked potato. However, the baked potato served here was quite different, and to be fair I did NOT generalize the American baked potato on the basis of that one experience at the hospital. I had shared the picture of it with friends and it was just that, one brown, shriveled potato looking lost, lonesome and sad, sitting all alone on a quarter plate! A small packet of neglected sour cream slouched on the tray next to it. The potato really didn't look cooked but on prodding with a fork we were happy to note that it was and our girl ate it while making a thousand comical faces with eyebrows raised. Presentation was clearly an art known to few. My neighbor Gina's views on baked potato were that it was comfort food for many in the States. I agreed, it did bring comfort with a smile

Just when we thought that Lavanya's chemotherapy schedule was progressing without unexpected complications, an unpleasant surprise came in the form of high blood sugar, another side effect of one of the drugs from the cocktail of drugs she was receiving for killing the leukemic cells. The interesting part was that the same drug might have the above reaction in one patient and not in another and sometimes on two separate occasions have different reactions on the same patient. One knew it only when the side effect happened, keeping surprise a constant factor. With high sugar she had to use the rest room more often, walking in pain and then pee in a hat, and excuse me I don't mean the one you wear on your head. The hospital hat is a plastic dispenser with ml markings, put on top of the seat so the nurses or caregivers may measure output against input. One learned as one went along, taking precautions from lessons learned in the past until the next surprise came. We began to monitor and measure carbohydrate intake against the insulin doses given prior to every meal, just another new aspect added to the expanding list of dos and don'ts. Lavanya showed extreme resilience as she happily offered her fingers to the nurses for checking the blood sugar and sometimes doing it on her own. The regimen continued for good two weeks while the effect of the medication went through her system leaving her without diabetes once it left.

At this juncture, with induction on, there were two schools of thoughts on her treatment plan. One school thought that she would be an ideal candidate for a bone marrow transplant from her younger brother, provided he matched. While the second school of thought recommended

43

the regular chemotherapy protocol reserved for all acute lymphoblastic leukemia patients. In their opinion the disease occurring after a decade could not be classified as a relapse. The decision was to happen after the first bone marrow test that was scheduled two weeks from the start of treatment and another test to check the Minimum Residual Disease (MRD) that could find one cancerous cell in a million normal cells. That would confirm her response to the treatment.

Meanwhile between her siestas, Varun and I caught up over Starbucks coffee in the cafeteria. I couldn't fathom as to why there was a craze for this concoction they called coffee. It was not drinkable and the description of sizes was confusing and misleading. I realized that small meant tall and grande was larger than tall, with venti being close to the largest. Okay, I admit I am a north Indian, basically a tea drinker and didn't enjoy my cuppa of coffee until we started living and loving it in Melbourne. Melbourne introduced us to an array of coffee that we had never heard of. We got the regular espresso, cappuccino and then there were the flat whites, short blacks and long blacks. I had associated long and black only with hair until then. The milk added a kick with choices of skinny milk, soymilk in Melbourne while America has its 1% and 2% fat milk in addition to the almond milk, soy milk and a lot more. So after Melbourne's quaint cafes, Starbucks with its gigantic serves of cappuccino paled in comparison. But then following the motto of when in Rome be a Roman, I say Starbucks was my lifeline while at the hospital and it was not bad to stand in that little queue, er line actually, at the Stanford Café where, as a frequent flyer, the person serving would always ask, "And how's your girl today?" as they gave me a 'wet coffee.' The ignorant me thought all coffee/liquids are wet! But then when we can drink dry wine, what's wrong with wet coffee! English sure is a funny language.

Talking of this miracle beverage coffee, I thanked God for all the McDonald meals we had eaten as the Ronald McDonald cart would come into the corridors distributing presents for the patients and coffee for the parents. So that little box at the cash counter does something remarkable for parents of cancer patients in addition to thoughtful gifts for all ages and gender getting therapy as admitted patients. They have something for that two-year-old across the corridor as well as something for our 15-year-old and the 17-year-old next door. I even drank that beverage they called coffee very gratefully as it saved me a trip to the cafeteria downstairs. Our Melbourne coffee maker would just faint with sheer disbelief that we were drinking that beverage. They were coffee snobs, on similar lines as wine snobs, calling themselves the coffee connoisseur but they meant well and their coffee was divine!

Meanwhile, Ditto, our eleven-year-old boy was perplexed as to what kind of a disease this was, having a high level of drug intervention and lengthy hospital stay. His exposure to diseases was limited to one missing school for a couple of days, a few coughs, some sniffles, a course of antibiotic or maybe a broken bone or at the most the yearly flu shot. On explanation and grasping most of it he quietly declared that he thought that his sister was the bravest person he knew. In my eleven-year old's words, "There is a battle inside her body between the good cells and the bad cells, with the good cells winning." I must admit that I was proud of my explanation as I heard his graphic description of the battle of the cells with the leukemia cells having a tremendous loss. There were sounds, lights and lots of special effects in his vivid description. I could almost visualize the cell war. Yes, he is a boy and a science fiction fan; only instead of Luke Skywalker it was Lavanya Rajpal, cell war replacing Star Wars. He did bring a smile onto the faces of all listening.

With aggressive therapy Lavanya's counts began to play see-saw with falling platelets, hemoglobin and WBC, requiring transfusion. The blood sugar, too, fell requiring adjustment of insulin, suddenly making a gigantic jar of orange juice a mandatory roommate. The big day was the next day as there was a scheduled bone marrow test with epidural anesthesia instead of general anesthesia. I recall her wanting to hold my hand as she fell asleep and I did my best to not cry looking at my child, seeming so small amidst all the instruments, gadgets, doctors and nurses. The doctors kept talking to her.

"Lavanya, what's your favorite place in the world?"

"My room."

"Where in your room?"

"My bed."

"What's there in your room?"

"Lots of pictures!"

"What else?"

"Mess on the floor ..."

And this went on until she fell asleep. So brave! So innocent! So trusting!

At Stanford for every needle poke, she received a bead, for every bone marrow test a special bead, for every transfusion very special beads. Strung together whenever time permitted, I was sure that she would make a beautiful necklace, a silent testimony of her endurance.

Then there dawned a morning which broke my heart some more, if it were possible, as I saw her staring at her pillow scattered with hair. However, to my surprise she giggled and cheered up, instructing me, "Tell grandma that I am going to be bald before her, eat many more medicines than she does, walk with help unlike her so I am an old lady and not grandma." My mother-in-law and she would often compare whose hair fell more, who ached more or who tired more easily and she was pleased to be able to boast that she was a winner there.

Chapter 6

"When you want something badly, the whole universe conspires to achieve it for you."
Ralph Waldo Emerson, Paulo Coelho and a few others

I believe many great people have said the above in different words. I had to use it on a beautiful spring day to report that the initial bone marrow test performed after fifteen days of treatment showed no leukemia cells and growth of new cells. She was officially in remission.

I couldn't thank God enough and each and every one in our little circle, our universe, that conspired to help attain the huge milestone making me feel that I could dance all night. When I shared this milestone on the blog, the number of phone calls and messages that followed moved me to tears. Some wanted to dance with me all night while others went to their respective places of worship to express their great big thank you to their Lord Almighty. I believe many had an impromptu party and rejoicing with family and friends. Our friends' families, friends and neighbors joined in the journey of remission by just hearing regularly about the teen who was a stranger to them. While I always believed that Lavanya would respond to treatment and recover well, her initial response strengthened that belief into conviction and I knew truly that this was just another test that would soon be behind us. I realized that with belief we have the ability to change our lives just as we are the makers of our destiny.

Stanford Children's Hospital has a school for their in-patients. It is heartwarming to be aware of the numerous aspects covered and the resources provided by the hospital to make a child's stay seem far from that of a grueling confining treatment. I did a little jig when I saw Lavanya walking after physical therapy all the way from the first floor to the third floor to attend school. The dragging of the IV pole with all its paraphernalia attached becoming a completely neglected and forgotten hindrance. On reaching there I am sure children felt akin to those present there as each child had attached tubes, some masked heavily signifying stem cell transplant patients, others with the lighter mask, most of them way too weak and battered by chemotherapy to do much, but welcoming that respite away from their rooms into a colorful sunny room with classroom atmosphere. Mums pushed some in wheelchairs, while some had their dads with them and then there were others with their grandparents. All had their best friend the IV pole faithfully standing next to them. I was grateful to note that patients with parents at work had volunteers helping them.

On return from the school we were met with the hospital teacher who came to see Lavanya and see her she did. She stared at her long and hard with a twinkle in her eyes, asking with a smile, "Who are you? You must be someone very special. I received the sweetest letter from your school saying we should not give you any work. They want to give you time to recuperate completely and they will help you to catch up when you go back. The hospital school does not have to keep you up to date with your class schedule. I have never seen this happening so your teachers must think very highly of you." Lavanya told her that the assistant principal Mr. Michael Hicks had called her after a meeting with all her teachers and they decided they would like her to concentrate on recovery and if she wanted work they would send her selective work depending on her wellness and capability. I had not heard of any other school, college or institution that were as involved, thoughtful and helpful.

Someone rightly said there is a silver lining somewhere; we just have to keep our eyes wide open. With the school management and staff being helpful beyond imagination, Lavanya focused solely on recovery rather than recovery along with catching up with academics. She set a goal for herself that come August she would attend school regularly, right from the first day after summer and spoke to her doctors about it. They looked at her and then at one another, finally looking at me. One of them quietly said, "Well, we have had patients diagnosed in April usually start school around Christmas!" Lavanya just gasped! Christmas was so far away and she would miss way too much. Her primary oncologist Dr. Lacayo intervened and put her mind to rest with, "Honey, if you think you can attend school from August and your counts are not too low, you will attend school from August." God bless this soft spoken gentleman who imbibed the faith that doctors so strive for and patient's family look for, some simply have it effortlessly while others despite pouring over management books never quite reach there. So she rested and the 'to-do list' just grew both in size and interest.

The assistant principal, councilor and teachers factored in aspects we had not known or thought of. Their foresight of graduation requirement, credits, deadlines, College Board policies had them meeting multiple times. Between them they devised a unique way Lavanya could complete her graduation requirement with home schooling once discharged and catch up with class when attending school. Chemotherapy induced neuropathy made walking and writing difficult so provision for more time as well as use of a word processor was allowed for her assignments and tests with written permission from the College Board. Since she was immuno-compromised they worked again with the College Board so she could write her SAT in isolation at her own school rather than one of the many centers with hundreds of others. She was given the option to use the school elevator but our warrior preferred to walk up holding onto the rails or with the help of friends. When I dropped her to school, there would be someone to help her with her bag if she needed help. One day I dropped her late to school after a round of chemo, a perfect stranger standing by the gate smiled at me and yelled in assurance, "Don't worry, we have her back!"

Mary Jane, from Melbourne wrote beautifully. Her thoughtfulness came onto paper/screen to warm anyone reading them. She wrote, "Dear Lavanya, we feel for you and all you are going through. Out of each day though, there has been great and miraculous news bringing tears of joy, hope and love from Australia. All our prayers are directed to you and your entire family and friends. After reading your mum's comments and summary of how your days have been, we have named you our young 'Aussie Trooper.' You push through each difficult day and come out with an amazing attitude and that sense of humor still shines. We send all our love and prayers from across the land and seas." Any surprise that I was in tears on reading this! Within moments of her post on the blog, my phone beeped with a WhatsApp message from Usha in Mumbai, "Who is Mary Jane? She writes so beautifully and echoes all our feelings. She really speaks for all of us." The global bonding between strangers was beginning.

When Lavanya developed agonizing pains in her back, she was advised a spine X-ray to check for compression on the spine and was wheeled into the X-ray department to be sent right back as the nurses at oncology had not included a negative pregnancy test result. Pregnancy test!!! Huh! Apparently hospital rules mandate that any female over the age of 10 must show a negative pregnancy test not more than a week old before being X-rayed. Lavanya, though, couldn't understand why the pregnancy test was required of inpatients who had barely any strength to move out of the room for close to a month, let alone have some romance. She laughed about it saying, "What do they expect!" Well,

I supposed that protocols were laid down for certain reasons and were required to be followed.

Back home the postman was kept busy as along with wishes and prayers, a lot of cards and presents, too, had been pouring in. She couldn't believe that parcels were coming from Melbourne, Singapore, India and nodded her head wisely with divine knowledge, sagely saying, "A sick child gets more presents than a birthday child."

With blood sugar in control, Lavanya tried Jhoomar's food and realized what she had been missing. Jhoomar is my childhood friend and neighbor who I discovered lived not 15 minutes' drive away. Suddenly the eyes opened wide and senses alert, Lavanya proclaimed – "No more hospital food!!" So dad made asparagus lemon risotto for our girl and brought it back. She polished it off and looked very pleased. Yes, it was delicious. I conveyed grateful thanks to Jhoomar, Mali and Gita for all the dabbas/tiffins.

Initially I separated all food boxes received from different sources. I put them in colored bags, red for Jhoomar, blue for Mali, green for Gita but all in vain. There was a huge confusion of the Tupperware, zip lock and all assortments of boxes and I thought I would throw a great big party where owners could enjoy a scavenger hunt to find their boxes from the huge lot. Of course the party didn't happen as there were many other developments, but most of the tiffins/boxes reached their rightful owners and the ones that didn't, well, now the owners know each other pretty well with the common agenda of, 'helping the Rajpals' binding them. They meet at various fund raising activities that Lavanya began for the Leukemia and Lymphoma Society so I was sure they could retrieve that lost tiffin if they really wished. The Mali I talk about is another childhood friend I discovered living five minutes away and coincidently our children go to the same school. Talk about a small world! Gita is Varun's colleague and friend, Ashwin's wife, and she drove a good one hour to provide us with regular delicious nutrition.

The spine X-ray reports showed that there was no compression so maybe the pain was caused by frequent lumbar punctures. Lavanya had that much desired bath finally with the bone marrow test dressing off. She looked like a new girl! Though she did comment, "Mommy, my face is so round and my legs have become like sticks. I look funny." We discussed that it was the steroid effect and would be temporary. She amusedly juggled her multiple chins but didn't look very pleased at the overall picture of balding head, chubby cheeks, jiggling chins and matchstick legs. I didn't know what to call her handling of the situation – mature or childlike, brave or that of an escapist or something else that I have no word for. I know mature people throwing a fit if something went wrong with their looks or body and similarly I have heard of children throwing tantrums if they didn't fancy what they were wearing or how they looked in a certain dress. Cancer doesn't make one beautiful, and it can only be the inner beauty and resilience that can shine from a body battered every other day with chemotherapy.

When the doctors and nurses kept telling Lavanya that she was being really good, she quipped, "It's easier to be good than bad." Universal truth really, but not tried often enough. Seriously if everyone tried being good they would realize how much effort and energy actually went in to be

54

difficult. We were expected to continue the sugar check once discharged so were given a practice kit for blood sugar test. We had been told to practice on ourselves for a while before we started testing Lavanya's sugar levels. I had not realized that I flinched every time Lavanya had her blood sugar tested. Imagine a sound like a stapler or even a punching machine jutting a needle into your child's thumb and fingers. Will you not flinch! She wanted to convince me that it really didn't hurt and went on, "Mommy you got to let me poke you once for blood draw to make you realize that it doesn't hurt." Lordy!!! Yep so I had my sugar tested, three pokes in three fingers to get the sufficient dot of blood on the strip. Varun and Lavanya were convinced that I was a vampire. It took forever to get my blood and it wasn't even blue, as I had proclaimed it would be. Neither a vampire nor royalty, how boring was that!

Chapter 7

*"When someone has cancer, the whole family
and everyone who loves them does, too."*

Terri Clark

With muscles weakening due to inactivity Lavanya was advised three short walks through the day to get blood flowing, with legs moving, arms swinging. During our walk around the corridors of Bass Center for Childhood Cancer and Blood diseases, we met other children with their buddy the IV pole on one side and mum, dad, aunt, uncle or grandparent on the other. We would exchange greetings, sharing the oft similar side effects and how each one was handling or managing the situation thrust upon them and wishing each other well. We would be saddened to hear of setbacks and rejoiced about improvement and recovery.

After one such walk as I went to the parent's kitchen to heat something, I was surprised to be greeted with exclamations of, "Oh there she is!" One mum gave me a hug and promptly I hugged her back. We exchanged our names, our children's names, grades, where each one was from and where we stood in the treatment. One had already completed a stem cell transplant, another was in a clinical trial; one was waiting for transplant with a ten on ten match from the sibling. They thought I was the lucky one whose child didn't need a transplant, but then they looked fearful at the knowledge that for us it was the second time, it had come back after ten years. Each one was of a different nationality, some traveling from another state, living in the Ronald McDonald House at Stanford and then there were the lucky ones like us who drove just 15 miles to get the treatment. One of the mums hesitantly told me, "I always look for you when you are coming and going because seeing you cheers me up." I was very touched that I could do that to a perfect stranger but I wondered aloud how that was possible. She said that the reasons were my pearls and my smile. Apparently I always wore pearls and I had to smile at that. Guilty as charged! I wear pearls with jeans, shorts, skirt, salwar kameez and saree. I wear them all the time, whether gardening, going to school or going to a party, whether am happy or am sad or in good times and bad times, the pearls are always there and most believed they helped in holding me up. Was it a surprise that soon we had many mums sitting in the parent's room of oncology floor all sporting different kinds, lengths and sizes of pearls, sipping coffee and chatting as though waiting at our children's school for them to emerge from classes. I called us the pearl brigade! They are part of me as much as the smile I wear which I guess comes from growing up in a family that had a fridge magnet saying, "You aren't dressed for the day until you wear a smile."

Basically, dressing well, wearing jewelry, behaving upbeat had a positive effect on the mind. If the body looked and felt fresh, the mind, too, couldn't be far behind. Think whatever suits you, getting off the right side of the bed, wearing a particular color, wearing a lucky dress or jewelry, because at the end of the day it's all in the mind. If we think something is going to work, nothing can stop it from working except probably our own mind. Call it superstition or solace, if a belief helps in achieving the goal it is a worthwhile belief as it creates faith followed by perseverance.

Soon parents knew which stage of therapy the other family was going through, how each child reacted to drugs, which drug was the easy one and which one everyone felt fearful about. When the families chatted, surprisingly we didn't talk about the child undergoing treatment. We always spoke as 'we' are now here for two weeks, 'we' are due for this particular drug or, 'we' are in the induction part of the treatment or even 'our' counts are low so 'we' are going to be here for a while.

Truly, the disease affects the patient and anyone who loves them. Our friends in different parts of the world would have goose bumps when 'we' suffered from painful side effects. They prayed more fervently when 'we' sounded low and celebrated when 'we' felt better. Just one member of the family living as a patient in the hospital tears a home apart. When the reason for being that patient is cancer and that too in your young child, the tear is not limited to home only but also extends to heart, mind and wellbeing of the entire family and friends.

Lavanya's friend Yana was a regular hospital visitor, a lovely Russian girl born on the same day as our girl and new to America just like her. I smiled as I overheard Lavanya telling Yana gleefully – "My mum is leaky you know!" I apparently leaked from my eyes and she found that funny! What else did she expect me to do! Sing and dance while she was in pain, though I did take care that she was not watching or awake, but clearly I had not succeeded.

Achala came up with an appropriate phrase, "Just plug the leaks, Sohini."

Achala, a dear friend in Melbourne to whom the assistant principal of the school introduced me to saying that he knew someone just like me, a family just like mine. I give the gentleman A plus on people perception as that was the beginning of a beautiful cherished friendship between the two families. Another friend, Usha, whose daughter and Lavanya have been friends since almost always, sent me texts the moment she was up and again before she slept. Just a little hey, what's on, am thinking of you, praying etc. She let me know that she was there praying hard and wishing well all the time. Through these people, I learned about lending support to others in difficult situations, realizing that it is not awkward to offer help and words of kindness or understanding. At worst you may be ignored but at best it would make a difference – a good kind of difference initiating a circle of giving.

Hikari, another friend of Lavanya's came by with stories of pig dissection in school that had us grimacing and laughing at the same time, though the animal activists might not be amused. A lovely delicate girl from Japan with a soft and humble diction, her rendition of the same was indeed memorable as she narrated in her low soft voice – "The pig's face looked so cute, but we had to cut it!!" When we were at school, and am talking of the 1980s, the maximum one came close to dissecting an animal was a frog. Lavanya had dissected a cow's eye and after that a sheep's heart in Melbourne. I loved hearing about the experiences of the students today; the journey has become tougher but more fascinating.

The next evening, I returned home to find a bag with pearl necklace dropped into the letterbox, thanks to Gina. She read the previous update of mums thinking wearing pearls was a good way of staying cheerful. She very thoughtfully bought beautiful pearls to be gifted to another mum, a woman unknown to her, to bring cheer, hope and normalcy in her life. What a fantastic gesture from one stranger to another! Rita, another buddy from Melbourne, felt convinced that the pearls would hold the mums up spreading good cheer. This Aussie lady was very impressed with the Americans who opened their doors and hearts to us in a very short time. So cheers to America with regards from Australia!

Another fantastic thing I discovered on returning home was that the dishwasher had been emptied, kitchen cleared, laundry done with clothes folded and ironed. What could bring more pleasure at any time of the day than to find all chores done? Clearly the magic lady Lubna had arrived! I feel marriages are made in heaven. Why I say that now, because 20 plus years of marriage has me loading dishwasher every night and Varun emptying it every morning. This has been happening with clockwork precision for two decades, without any discussion or agreement whether written or oral. We didn't write a prenup on anything! We hadn't made a list of chores to divide between us; this was an unconditional understanding without discussion. With hospital stays divided between the two of us, things like dishwasher, washer, dryer, groceries, etc., were done by whoever was home for a longer duration and some days even our Ditto took on the chore.

With Lubna's arrival these seemingly small but unavoidable chores were taken over completely by her. I didn't have to hold her hand through an introduction to the kitchen and found her dishing out meals as though she cooked there every day! She took over Ditto's homework schedule, too, as if she had been doing it forever and spent some nights at the hospital so Varun and I could stay home together with Ditto. He was thrilled with both parents home all for him, and Lavanya was delighted with the undivided attention of aunty Lubna. We thought we were blessed with a beautiful family and thanked God for the same. We have no choice as regards family, we are born into it and then they are born to us, but with friends it's a miracle to find that person with who you connect in mind and spirit.

Usha felt that it was very nice of us to appreciate every small magical moment but then I thought it was so much easier to appreciate than to complain. It came with an added benefit of a feel good factor to those appreciating as well as those appreciated. I thought we were the lucky ones, else how could these magical things happen amidst all the hiccups. I thanked God that we could recognize the magic because surely, there was a possibility of it passing by without us acknowledging it.

Another beautiful surprise came in the form of a lovely quilt made by our very talented and creative neighbor Anita and her Church's quilting group. What a treasure! It was soft, beautiful and one could feel the love and best wishes it was made with; our girl was truly wrapped in God's love.

The doctor dropped by to share that the Minimum Residual Disease or MRD test results from the 15th day bone marrow test showed that the disease was less than 0.00001 per 100,000 cells. MRD was not available a decade back in India and it has been a boon to leukemia treatment because it could measure the smallest level of cancer cells in tissue samples. It could find one leukemia cell in a million normal cells revolutionizing the understanding of the disease; its extent, remission possibilities, thereby aiding the selection of protocol to achieve complete remission. I felt this was possible so quickly only because the universe conspired. We were told that if the day 29 Bone Marrow Test (BMT) and Minimum Residual Disease (MRD) looked any similar to the day 15 of treatment, she would continue the normal leukemia treatment of approximately three years, ruling out a stem cell transplant. We had no way of conveying what we felt, so we just held each other quietly thanking God and our Universe.

The song dance and honeymoon period was cut short by a night of terrible pains, requiring not one but two IV injections of morphine followed by sedative. Of course Lavanya, still the ever inquisitive teen had one more query before the drug kicked in totally, "Hey mommy, check how

I sleep and tell me if I wake up exactly like this the next time I wake up so we will know how the medicine knocks me out, if I move at all in my sedated sleep." On that excitement she slept and got up in almost the same posture.

Painkillers were administered every six hours and more X-rays were ordered to check ankle, back and knees. Lavanya's chiropractor, Lisa, dropped by and the two chatted like buddies meeting after a long time. I thank Google for having Lisa in our lives. When Lavanya's back was giving her issues I had looked on Google for a chiropractor in our area and that was the beginning of a great doctor patient relationship as well as friendship with her.

Beginning the fourth week of our hospitalization the doctors said that they were thinking of a discharge as her WBC, platelets and hemoglobin looked good. Imagination is a wild gift of God. The moment someone said the WBCs were looking good I imagined well made up white blood cells looking prim and proper, behaving themselves. I thought of a group of platelets doing what they are supposed to be doing with diligence.

In anticipation of discharge, tutorials to take care of Lavanya and her PICC line at home began for Varun and me. Our respect for high school students, in fact for all students increased many folds as we sat through three back-to-back study/training sessions of more than three hours. We were also taught with a dummy on how the port would be placed on her chest with a small surgery after the PICC line removal. This would be the point from where all her treatment, labs would be done in future. Port is a very small plastic or metallic disc that is inserted just under the skin with a tube connecting it to a prominent vein. Port could be accessed by specialized needle of different sizes depending on the patient and this ended the search for thin, elusive veins and multiple needle pokes.

Lavanya wondered and couldn't understand why many adults talked to her about her hair loss, how did it warrant a conversation every time! According to her it would grow back, probably better so she was not concerned. In fact, this time she intended to make a style statement with scarves. I suggested shaving designs on her head when little hair started growing back. We thought of having a poll later to ask for suggestions on multiple ways to wear scarves or how to shave an amazing design on a fresh crop of hair. And then what happened? United States Postal Services was kept very busy delivering scarves from Asia, Australia and Europe to our doorsteps.

The Make a Wish foundation people approached Lavanya to make a wish and she expressed her wish to go to France. Varun came up with ideas like wishing for a meeting with Shah Rukh Khan, Daniel Radcliff or Emma Watson. Sorry to say that the celebrities didn't impress her. Though now two years on she says she could have thought of requesting to meet Emma Watson, as she is most impressed with this young actor who is Goodwill Ambassador at the United Nations. The make a wish people said one boy wanted to go to Italy and did just that, another watched soccer game in South Korea, smaller kids loved a visit to Disneyland so it all depended on what the child really wanted and not what the parents thought was appropriate. Varun and I told her to wish for something simpler as there were a lot of kids and some in very unfortunate circumstances and the family could make a trip later once she was better. We were told by The Make a Wish official that we were not to interfere in the wish making process with any suggestions. Their explanation was very simple that when a child has cancer; the whole family goes through the treatment and ordeal, so when the child wished for something, the whole family got it.

Chapter 8

"Grief is in two parts. The first is the loss.
The second is the remaking of life."

Anne Roiphe.

With diagnosis on 26th March 2013, we were discharged exactly 24 days later. It was the most beautiful drive and the most cherished sight was Ditto waiting for us, opening the car door and escorting his sister in, all the while holding her hand. I remembered the hymn we learned as children, 'Count your blessings, name them one by one, and you will be surprised what God has done.' When we begin to count, we realize that the list can be endless. Priya Devotta, my buddy from high school teared up on reading the counting of blessings and remembered hearing her grandma saying the same but that as a mum she could appreciate the value of the saying aptly.

One evening I overheard Varun talking to someone on phone in very chaste Hindi, explaining that all was well. It turned out to be the driver from 'Autoriders Mumbai' who drove him around during his business trips to India. The company attempts to send the same car and driver every time, so the driver had his entire schedule. Since there was a break the last time, with Varun cutting short his trip to return home, the driver had enquired and Varun had explained. That guy, that so sweet guy called from Mumbai to check if all was well every few days giving his assurance that he was praying and wishing us all well. Can one even imagine that!! An everyday cab driver concerned about the wellness of his not so regular passenger's daughter. I say again, the world is beautiful, abundant with wonderful people. I do sound repetitive but I couldn't stress enough on what we learned through our diagnosis and treatment, we just need to keep our eyes and ears open to find beauty around us.

The delight of the return of the daughter home was shared worldwide, own room, own bed, messy floor and no hat to pee. I could just walk over to her room to see her either sleeping soundly or staring at us with big beautiful eyes. Often Varun would stay up telling her favorite childhood story. Some of them were hilarious then and are more so now, as then to a five-year-old they seemed to make a whole lot of sense and now a decade later I think she just liked the sound of her dad's voice going up and down. I must admit that I too loved the sound of his voice going up and down, saying the same story every time year after year. The man doesn't know too many! The oft repeated story told since birth goes something like this, once upon a time in a faraway land there was a place called Mumbai. In Mumbai there was a place called SEEPZ (The Santa Cruz Electronics Export Processing Zone). In SEEPZ there was a company called CITIL (Citicorp Information Technologies Industries Ltd) and it went on and on with the people in the company traveling all over the world, meeting new people, working with different people, seeing new places etc. It did make a fascinating story. Sometimes Varun's visiting friends would add a twist to the story by introducing technical terms like 'Linux' etc.

Lavanya felt that medical science was confusing. With rough days due to multiple medications, one causing nausea, the other causing constipation, something making her gain tremendous weight and something else making her lethargic – medical science was indeed confusing. She had nausea troubling her when lying down and fatigue dampening her when up. 105 mg of steroids a day caused havoc in her system and the poor thing felt the weight of her cheeks too heavy to allow her to talk. Not yet 18 but she took 18 tablets of various sizes and shapes daily. Varun cut some and crushed the others to fill in a hollow capsule to not only mask the dirty taste but also to reduce the numbers. This was over and above the pain and nausea medication as and when required.

A very confused Lavanya said, "First I am given medication to fix something, then another medication to correct what the previous medication unfixed and this goes on! Why couldn't there be a solitary medication that does right without doing any wrong." We await the day this will happen – a one pill cure for cancer or a vaccination just like the measles, flu shot. I am happy to visualize all

68

Pharmacy's board in 2020 saying- flu shots, meningitis shots, cancer shots, available.

We received the very sad news of the passing away of Varun's colleague and friend Scott Dawes's high school going son, a lovely boy, to cancer in Melbourne. I recall him joining the Mother's Day run during remission. Such a brave wonderful boy! We all prayed for the beautiful soul gone too early and for the family. This made us wish and want that cure for cancer soon, so no more young lives are lost. We were touched to read condolence messages pouring in for Scott Dawes's son, Connor, from all our friends. Everyone wished the family strength, hope and prayed for the young soul to rest in peace. The beauty of human nature was evident again. None of the people who had expressed their thoughts in the blog about Scott's son knew either him or the boy, but everyone felt the loss of a young life, someone's son, a brother, a nephew and a friend.

Trying to think very practically, in the circle of life, the loss of a parent is inevitable with age. But one wouldn't like to live the day to lose a child, that's an endless vacuum, immortalized with all love, each thought, every breath, every day while life went on. We, too, prayed for the family and it is now three years since the irreplaceable loss, and the family has already made great inroads in keeping the memory of their beloved first-born alive beyond their circle of family and friends. The RCD Foundation, (Robert Connor Dawes) is a foundation established in Melbourne, Australia to battle brain tumor and support brain matters in areas of research, development and care. I doff my hat to this family and their supporters. It is simple to close ourselves with and in grief. It is very easy to drift with the same grief, in depression, create animosity, seclusion, broken homes and live a life of a cynic with hate and anger. Life of a victim is probably easier to lead than the life of inspiration – to take matters in your own hands, stand united, create, inspire, spread love and faith despite that gaping hole in your heart are sum total of things no book can teach. I feel honored to be in the circle of this family who have done much in the memory of their boy and taught everyone the capability of channeling grief and energy in a direction that changed and continues to change many lives. They simply multiplied the love for their boy and I believe they call it productive grief. They remade and immortalized their boy with the strength of their mind and love in their heart by establishing a fund that continues to support brain matters. And he will live on till eternity.

Chapter 9

"The power of community to create health is far greater than any physician, clinic or hospital."
Mark Hyman

Many people are allergic to nuts, some to eggs, some to gluten, some are lactose intolerant and some react to certain antibiotics. Now Lavanya is special, she has allergy to blood! I guess she preferred only her own but then that lifesaving blood has been transfused so many times since treatment began that every time I see a unit getting into her, I thank all those strangers, the unknown people in this world who go all out and donate blood to save lives, lives of people they don't know, aren't aware of their existence. I sent those strangers whose blood now runs in our girl's veins silent thanks and continue to bless them every day.

This allergy was discovered at the time of her first transfusion when her heart rate shot up to 150 beats a minute with breathlessness, as soon as the transfusion began. The protocol for such circumstances was immediate oxygen intervention with transfusion interrupted until a cause was identified. With the allergy known there was always pre-medication, followed by very slow transfusion.

Lavanya was on schedule for surgery for removing the PICC line and placement of port. Prior to the procedure she was required to get a good wash and she sat in the bath as I gave her a wash while we chatted quietly. The chat included general mundane things as if life was normal, none betraying the fact that we were preparing for a surgery to mark the beginning of a long grueling treatment, until she groaned. She moaned and groaned, "Oh mommy, this is so hard!" My heart went out to her, almost leaking from my eyes, dripping from my nose, I hugged my wet girl and spoke about that being one of the tough phases of the treatment and how well she had coped. She groaned louder, "Mother!! The stool I am sitting on is hard." Aha, duh me!

Our friends found Lavanya's tongue in cheek humor infectious. Priya in Mumbai drove to Shirdi to worship and Priya from Delaware went off to church to offer her prayers while Alka began chanting with her Buddhist group. Radhika initiated a Facebook prayer group. By then the regular commentators for my updates had become virtual friends holding each other in high esteem. Achala was grateful that someone like Lisa was by our side and expressed her desire to meet her someday. Usha in Mumbai was amazed by the support of my school friend Shilpi in Singapore. Most had become huge fans of Mary Jane and echoed her words to me. These complete strangers formed a common bond and developed mutual respect. Lavanya's friend Valli wrote that school seemed a bit boring. Madame Finck, their French teacher talked about her to them every day at lunch and all of them missed her. They got together at lunch to read the blog and updated those who were not a part of it. It had served its purpose and I didn't have to answer the phone all day repeating the same information over and over again.

As we waited in pre-op Lavanya made some observations. She was tired but had to share her newly acquired wisdom. She whispered about similarities of a developed nation America with that of a so-called developing one or even third world nation India. Having spent good amount of time in the best hospitals of both the nations, the conclusions were pretty interesting. Common factors were that food sucked in all hospitals, nurses loved to party by talking and laughing loudly in both countries. They were generally a jovial and happy lot. If everything written in English is followed by its Spanish translation in California, in Mumbai it is Marathi. So there were no differences between nations, cities or maybe the hospitals of the cities. She looked weak, small and fatigued by the chemotherapy, lying in bed waiting to be wheeled into the OR and back from the surgery she continued to be in an anesthesia induced slumber as my thoughts traveled back and forth unable to hold onto the past but finding it difficult to concentrate on the present.

The incision continued to pain and laying down or getting up would stretch the stiches compounding the pain. While we helped her up and down, she joked that, now she knew what Akbar, the great Emperor and King felt, always holding his head very high. She needed to hold her head really high with the chins and cheek getting in the way. She asked me when she was older if we could buy lots of toys, soft toys and join the make a wish foundation or a similar organization to cheer up all those sick kids in the hospital. Her words – "You could be like the old volunteers who go from room to room showing pictures of their children when they had leukemia and current pictures when they are grown up with children of their own. Only difference would be that I, too, would like to accompany you." I reminded her that's what we did in Mumbai, too, when she recovered. Shilpi, too, recalled that when Lavanya was little we did similar trips in a Mumbai hospital, a little seven-year-old girl going very confidently from bed to bed to kids aged 2 to 14 talking, laughing, coloring and reading. The doctor in Lilavati Hospital was impressed with our girl and had asked us if we would mind visiting other children in various stages of the treatment. We would drive directly from school to the hospital, Lavanya still in her blue pinafore uniform, struggle to find parking in or around the hospital, get visitor's pass and meet a number of children, most struggling with side effects but the one common factor binding them in one bright circle was the courage and resilience they all reflected. Really, we adults were so ill at ease under the circumstances that it did take a kid to teach us normal reactions at such times. Lisa felt Lavanya was sweet, strong and droll and loved her insights, observations and humor and I agreed. It is not easy to think of others when a constant onslaught of pain and discomfort create problems in daily living. I was glad that she thought of it herself, proving that the outside support made a

74

difference to her, inspiring her to make similar positive difference.

Chapter 10

"The life so short, the craft so long to learn."

Hippocrates

The end of induction brought fewer medicines; highlight being the 105 mg of daily steroid stopped. Often after chemo we would be stuck in peak hour traffic and at those times our Aussie trooper would be in tears with pain, discomfort and nausea. I would park the car and Ditto not knowing how to help his wailing sister would pat her head and help us to tuck her in. One evening back at home, fatigued after a long difficult day in the hospital, I saw him looking mightily pleased with himself when he joined us for dinner. Varun peeped in to check on Lavanya and discovered the reason for his glee. Sitting next to her pillow was his favorite bright yellow angry bird soft toy. Oh the sacrifices of the siblings!

After a month in hospital she had arrived at some deductions. There were three kinds of doctors – first there were those who came into the room, talked and treated the 15-year-old like a toddler, concentrating on medical terms and went away. The second kind walked in, ignored the 15-year-old on the bed and talked to the parents and went away, the third and the ideal doctors are the ones who walked in, chatted with both parents and the patient normally, discussed everything from disease to school to the weather, time permitting, or else stuck to necessities and went away. It was interesting, amusing and at times exasperating to see full grown adults with the greatest qualifications following their names, treat a teenager like a toddler or ignore her altogether. Probably to some, being the third kind, the ideal kind came naturally just like Lavanya's two oncologists. They were God's gift to humankind. Probably the qualities came with age, experience or maybe because they were parents themselves. They had learned the craft and the skills that were needed in a compassionate and competent doctor. Dr Lacayo and Dr Dahl had been angels in disguise. The patience and the enthusiasm with which they talked to our girl about everything from the disease, its side effects to English literature, American history, British history, France, French language, culture, AP Environmental Science experiments or plain and simple SATs and how to ace them was very gratifying. They were both incredible, heartwarming and great listeners. She consulted them on her subject selection for grade 12. She wondered whether to take British literature or Advanced Placement Literature most commonly known as Brit Lit or AP lit in American high schools. They seemed to enjoy discussing the challenges of an AP (Advanced Placement) subject as against her love for British literature. While one doctor felt that she didn't need to prove anything to anyone by taking a large load, the other felt that she might enjoy the challenge. They agreed to monitor her chemo doses through her exams and SATs so she would be able to write to her best capabilities. Some of the drugs produced so much neuropathy in her fingers and toes that she couldn't hold a pen for the next few days or walk properly and at times even the use of her jaws to eat a decent meal was painful. She would be on liquid or semi solid diet until the jaw pain receded. Every time she had an exam, they understood her wish to do well despite the hindrance some of the drugs created for her by way of chemo fog and neuropathy. They worked around her will and wish with the best in medicine, to give her a life beyond cancer. When college acceptance and rejections started coming in, they told her that the rejections were not rejections but places she would not fit in. When they saw the list of colleges she was accepted into they marveled at her hard work, dedication and perseverance against the odds, so much so that they promised they would work with her so she could do her best academically just as she wished.

From time to time they did gently remind her, "Honey, you do realize you have had cancer twice and we don't want it to come back, so we do need to treat you within the limits your body can take."

I was surprised when Dr. Lacayo phoned himself, as he didn't want to wait on the good news over the weekend to tell the parents of Lavanya that her MRD results had arrived and there were no leukemia cells seen. There was absolutely no need for him make that call, the news could have waited while we held our breaths over the weekend. It mattered to him and he knew the news would make all the difference to the parents. Lavanya couldn't understand the yet again 'leaky mum!'

"Mommy, you are so funny – you cry when you are sad and now you cry when you are happy! I don't understand you, mommy."

I told her it took a mommy to understand another or even a daddy or aunts or uncles or friends. The news was shared and it felt like a job well done by all, starting with our girl for her endurance, her doctors for their craft and knowledge, her nurses for their competent care and to our circle of friends for their prayers and support. It takes a village to make a person after all!

Wherever in the world were the friends of Rajpals, song, dance and celebration followed the news of MRD result. At home though the rejoicing were cut short by agonizing pains in the leg. One moment we rejoiced only to request for worldwide prayers the next as our relief was cut short with agonizing pains exactly a month from her first visit to Stanford on diagnosis. On phoning her doctors we were summoned into emergency. We were told that sometimes when high doses of steroids were stopped suddenly those pains may occur 'in teenagers especially.' I did wonder why not reduce the doses in steps in the first instance without waiting to find out the hard way. In ER doctors administered three doses of morphine but that didn't ease the pain, more combinations of pain medication were administered through the IV and finally after 8 hours in ER she had some relief. The steroid was resumed with plans to reduce doses over the week. She required re-admitting for pain management but pediatric oncology didn't have any bed available so pediatric cardiology took her in. Till then I had been thinking that there were too many kids with cancer, but suddenly it looked like there were equal or more children in the cardiac unit.

The story of reaching the ER, too, had its moments. I had taken Ditto for community service for science project when Varun phoned saying that Lavanya didn't look good at all and he had called the oncologist on call only to have been summoned to the ER at the earliest. I didn't know anyone at the event and looked around worried because I couldn't pull him out while the event was on, but I needed to leave too. A very perceptive lady saw my predicament and asked me what was bothering me as I spoke to Ditto to stay put while I went home and returned to pick him up. When this unknown lady heard me, she took matters in her hands and shooed me out with the promise to drop our boy home when done. A perfect stranger came to our rescue! Ditto returned happy after finishing his scheduled project, quite at ease with this lady who turned out to be a classmate's mum. In days when one teaches the kids not to talk to strangers or go anywhere with them, this lady reinforced our faith in those strangers.

We had a meeting with our primary oncologist Dr Lacayo and nurse practitioner and the team to discuss the treatment thereon. Going forward Lavanya would be given regular ALL (Acute Lymphoblastic Leukemia) chemotherapy treatment without radiation or stem cell transplant. Leukemia has many variants, the most common being Acute Lymphoblastic Leukemia (ALL), Acute Myeloid Leukemia (AML), Chronic Myeloid Leukemia (CML) and Chronic Lymphocytic Leukemia (CLL). In addition to these four there are many others including the strangely named hairy cell leukemia. Acute Lymphoblastic Leukemia again has subtypes, B cell and T cell, Lavanya's being B cell. Her treatment protocol was chemotherapy over two and half years to three years depending on her tolerance levels, hemoglobin levels, cell counts, etc. Initial months would see her receiving intense chemotherapy with frequent infusions and high dose medicines tapering down towards the last eighteen months that would be the maintenance phase. If the initial response continued, there was no reason for a transplant and she was told that she could be cured again.

The doctor apologized saying that the only issue would be in the far future when she was expecting a baby, she would need to consult a cardiologist in addition to a gynecologist as the medications were known to weaken the heart muscles. She would undergo Echo Cardiogram before and after that particular medicine was administered to keep a check on her heart. The more I heard and conferred with her doctors the more I respected them. I felt that was a wonderful way to convey to her and the family that all will be fine and normal despite the aggressive therapy. A possible side effect of stem cell transplant and aggressive chemotherapy is known to be infertility. He answered all her queries with great patience, her wish to join school and attend regular classes. Was it ironical or was it sad that all this child wanted to do was attend regular school and yet she couldn't do something as simple and as taken for granted as that!

Chapter 11

Being at a cancer clinic with regularity opens multiple facets of life encountering different mindsets and people most of which would leave us feeling grateful for what we had – leukemia. It does sound strange that I was thankful for leukemia. I was grateful that we didn't have a recurring brain tumor or an inoperable cancerous tumor. Strangely that is what a mum told me as we discussed our diseases, "You are so fortunate that yours has leukemia, mine has brain tumor and it keeps coming back." My heart went out to the mum as she continued that her younger one felt so neglected that she broke the TV in a rage and I thought of our Ditto – a sixth grader, riding back from school to an empty home, heating food in a microwave, playing a bit and then starting homework, trying to complete everything before mum or dad returned from hospital. All the while he kept me updated by text messages which went like, leaving for home, reached, ate, starting homework, have a question in math, when are you back and so on and so forth. Some days I would receive a picture showing a stack of clothes he folded, while on others a picture of the dishwasher he emptied graced the screen of the phone. His sense of responsibility would kick in, to be the man of the house alongside dad, our very own responsible little man, all of 11 years of age. I teared up thinking of him as he sometimes tucked Lavanya into bed with his angry bird soft toy or giving me a hug or a kiss when I looked low. I thanked God for him, what an angel we have, for his understanding, his patience and his quiet acceptance of the huge change in his life, despite all our attempts to keep things normal. His kind of attitude of rising up to every occasion can't be taught or understood by reading books – it comes from within. Every time I think of his talks I have to smile to myself. When he was all of seven years of age he had looked at me with much love declaring that when he grew up he would build/buy a big house. He didn't like the idea that while his sister and he had their own rooms, mum and dad had to share one! He would buy a house that would give mum and dad their own separate rooms! Oh okay, umm Ditto, I stifled a laugh murmuring that I loved his thoughtfulness but I also loved sharing the room with dad.

Talking of attitudes our girl decided that she didn't like the after-effects of general anesthesia and hence would try the spinal chemo without it. She compared it to her math test in Melbourne where one was allowed to refer to a cheat sheet if required. She said, "Let the anesthetist be the cheat sheet." So the anesthetist stayed there in the room on standby – a very live experienced competent cheat sheet. It all went off well with partial sedation. Mum was sent off, of course with precision just before the insertion of needle. It took a lot of strength of the mind and soul to get a needle inserted into your spine without anesthesia. Even as I write I get goose bumps as I can't stop from picturing her curling by tucking knees to chest, in preparation for the procedure. I just might have leaked at an inappropriate time, though I do wonder if there is an appropriate time ever!

Lisa promised her pumpkin love soup again which she made with organic pumpkin, apple, garlic, tomato and lots of love so the name pumpkin love soup. After the chemo the first thing our girl did was call dad and ask, "What are you cooking for me today?" Dad must have mumbled something like your wish my command, ma'am, because on return we found the best Italian in California - 'mangia bene' - Italy straight on our plate made with much effort by him. Lavanya, Ditto and I decided that the best Italian that we had eaten in California was from dad's kitchen and not the renowned California Pizza Kitchens. Lavanya and Varun are perfectionists. They follow a recipe to the letter while I make do with what I have. I don't aim for perfection like them and hence never achieve perfect result. Some of the Jamie Oliver cuisine Varun replicated just made us wish to continue savoring the presentation on plate very slowly to make it last. Lavanya too ate slowly savoring every yummy bite, though for her it was a problem to chew and swallow, nothing gourmet about it.

I had to write Shilpi's words verbatim – "Tell Lavanya, am heavily addicted to coca cola. I managed to decrease my consumption of coke, but found it very difficult to give up on coke zero. In a week of excellent self-control, I would have one-two a week. After reading that she refused general anesthesia and gave the comparison with the Math cheat sheet, I was so overwhelmed by her wisdom, maturity and strength that I thought, me! 'Chaalis saal ki buddhi (40 years old woman),' crying over giving up coke! Tell her I have not touched one diet or zero coke since then. She is indeed my inspiration." When I read the above to Lavanya, she smiled, "Mum, please tell Shilpi aunty to drink not one but two cokes today, one for her and one for me. Once in a while it is actually good to do something you consciously gave up doing." Hmmm some teen logic!

At times having to spend hours waiting for her turn to get therapy or transfusion, we would walk around and on bad days she would sit on a wheel chair while I pushed her to do hospital tourism, exploring the long corridors lined with art, flower arrangements, kids' paintings and most of all we did people watching. We watched mums and dads with their children in various stages of the treatment. Most wore the same expression of faith, hope and belief. Some looked gaunt and tired while others looked as though they were in any place but the hospital. It was quite funny and heartening to note that whomever we had fleetingly known in the past month would stop and make small conversation. Most common thread would be, "Lavanyaaa, your hair hasn't fallen completely! What are you doing? You look amazing!" As the days turned into months and the hair fell off, eyebrows and lashes disappeared, steroids made the cheeks bulge with weight, the very same people would stop and say, "Hey your hair has finally fallen! It will come back! But you look cute with the cap/scarf." And in case of no headgear it would be, "Don't you want to wear a scarf or a cap honey?" If she were well enough to be walking they would say, "Oh Lavanyaaa you are walking! How lovely you look!" And if she was found on the wheel chair, "Oh honey, get well soon! Though you don't look too bad really." I do feel like adding a smiley after this. Everyone meant well and tried so hard to make her laugh through all the pain and discomfort! In the corridors of the hospital, everyone we encountered reflected attitudes of optimism, hope and encouragement.

We reached a stage where one drug needed to be administered every day for four consecutive days. The doctors and staff suggested that they would teach me how the same could be administered at home, thereby saving the drive as well as wait time.

Driving to hospital every day during intense therapy was an ordeal as immense fatigue and nausea were just some of the smaller issues. Chemo at home did entail Lavanya returning home accessed with the one-inch needle sticking out of the port on her chest. I didn't fancy the thought of administering chemo to my daughter but kept quiet for the greater good it would entail. Moreover, I reminded myself, was I not married to the most competent of men! He would administer the chemo! I called it the perfect delegation of work. I have done surgery wound dressing for my mum after her mastectomy so it was not that I was turned off by the sight of wound, blood, and gore, but somehow the thought of pushing chemo drugs into my child, whose beautiful eyes looked at me trustingly, egging me on, come on mommy you can do it, was just not my idea of being mommy.

Thank God for the daddy – my rock! I had been taught how to de-access the port so we could avoid a drive to the hospital just for the sake of de-accessing. As the nurses develop confidence in the capability and understanding of the parents they are happy to teach a few tricks to make life simpler. I, in turn showed how to de-access to Varun by inserting the one-inch needle into a pillow and pulling it out by snapping the butterfly like sides. It was not really rocket science but again, just like my inability to push medication into her, I couldn't imagine pulling out a one-inch needle from her chest. I have known husbands/dads to faint at the sight of blood and mums to hyperventilate when their children have been diagnosed with myopia, prescribed glasses or bleeding from minor wounds. I had nothing against them but I justified to myself that I was not overreacting.

The chemo at home turned out to be interesting and unexpected. Dad administering the drug into the IV with the mum reading instructions and handing over everything chronologically were expected; the unexpected was the patient to whom it was being administered. What was she doing? She was singing! Yes, she sang rhymes, French rhymes, sometimes in tune, sometimes off key, along with the English version just so the ignorant parents were aware. Does anyone realize that many rhymes have a common tune and scale? She was quite loud and seemed very happy. I wondered if the drug cytarabine that was being administered have a happiness quotient to it.

Ditto returned from school carrying a beautiful collage made by his teachers and class with origami flowers, pictures, cut outs and beautiful messages for speedy recovery. Apparently they spoke about Lavanya in class and other children came forward to speak about their experiences with cancer. Someone's mother had completed breast cancer treatment; someone's dad was going for regular checkup after therapy completion, a grandma or a grandpa, an uncle and an aunt. Cancer strikes everywhere. Ditto wasn't alone in his class. He shared what was happening at home with his teachers so they were aware of most day-to-day updates from him as well as my blog. It was very thoughtful of them to organize the collage and make Lavanya feel special.

Chapter 12

"Genuinely good people are like that.
The sun shines out of them. They warm you right through."
Michael Morpurgo

There was this week during the treatment when it was all quiet, peaceful with nothing happening. No chemo, no blood draw, no transfusion so much so that I didn't even drive the car out of the garage. And then I received a couple of worried texts, phone calls asking, "Sohini, all well? No update?" So I had to send out an update cheering, applauding digitally and appreciating all who stood by us through the ordeal with their prayers, best wishes, concern and comments. I had to immediately rush to the computer to set their worried minds to rest, to say that it had been a nice day. Lavanya slept through most of it WITHOUT painkillers! I had thought of adding this to the update the following day but brought it ahead just to celebrate and acknowledge the day, its beauty in its routine. I took the opportunity to thank everyone for being there, watching the blog, following it diligently, praying and wishing our girl well. And to her for her resilience, her humor despite adversity, her enthusiasm and being just, well, a good patient. I knew I was blessed.

Years ago when my sister and I took turns to nurse our mum back from cancer she was one of those few adults who was an amazing patient. And now my daughter, a strong child, who told her school friends interviewing her for a chemistry project, "Ask my mum all the tech stuff about the treatment. I just know what's happening to me, what I am feeling. Mum takes care of the tech stuff." Well, I never! For once I was called tech savvy while more often I felt like a tech retard, or let's make it sound better and say tech novice.

There were often days when on opening the front door, we would find a bag or a box or a tiffin. These usually contained, you guessed it, food. But many a time they were accompanied with magazines, book and prints of new therapies for leukemia researched by friends. At one time we found movie tickets to the latest kids flick running in town, for Ditto to go to with a friend. Mali had thoughtfully bought two tickets so our boy could go with a friend. Depending on the cuisine, we would guess who was the mysterious friend responsible for feeding us. Things like zucchini bread were definitely from Anita next door, Karen was the one with some amazing pastas. We attributed all south Indian delicacies to Mali, while Namrata was the unsurpassed queen of the Indian bread called paratha and Lisa was responsible for all the exotic soups coming our way. We were pretty proud of the fact that we always guessed right. Some didn't stay anonymous and left a note. Sometimes self-written poems or quotes worthy of the occasion were found. Expressions of support showed in so many ways at our door step became a learning experience for us. I promised myself that anyone needed that support I would go that extra step and inculcate all that we received, continuing the circle of joy of giving.

One day during labs at the hospital we were engaged in general chat with the nurse and I said to her that her accent sounded familiar. She said, "Oh I am a New Zealander, have you been there?" Small world! We told her that we had moved from Australia and she wanted to know from where. When we said Melbourne her smile just got wider with, "Oh I, too, lived in Melbourne, my daughter was born at the Royal Women's Hospital and I worked at the Royal Children's Hospital."

Then, of course, stories of nursing in Australia as compared to America, the Aussie accent, etc., followed, and by the time we left she had given us supplies: 'port needle' for my purse in case we got into an emergency and someone not from oncology had to access her port – we could be ready with the right size needle which worked for Lavanya. All the way home I thought, Aussie Aussie Aussie oye oye oye. The connection from down under built a bond that day.

I think about human nature; how funny it is in its predictability. We believed in positive thinking and its far-reaching effects, but one morning when we got a call saying that our primary oncologist Dr Lacayo wanted to meet us, how did I react (instinctively)? I went practically,

"OMG! Why does he want to see us! What's up? What could have gone wrong?" Why didn't I think that he wanted to catch up, say hello, how are you all? My doubts and fears were put to rest when I realized that all the good doctor wanted to do was to make us feel cared for and comfortable as he had not seen us for a while personally. Talking of OMG, I realized that we use so much abbreviations in our text talk that the other day in the supermarket, I read the nutrition label 0mg as OMG and for a second was nonplussed to see 'oh my god' on nutrition label until better sense prevailed.

The first stop while going to the hospital was at the boom gate to get the parking ticket from Les Smith, one of the regular security personnel who always had a big smile and a kind word. In fact, with people like him at the entrance, driving into the hospital everyday didn't feel daunting. He was just one of the many people who made the whole hospital experience memorable and trauma free. The one last place one wants to feel familiar, recognize or be recognized is a hospital and as days passed by that's what was happening. Right from the individuals who manned the entrance boom gate, valet parking staff, reception staff, doctors, nurses, therapists down to the cafeteria staff, were all friends of Lavanya's mum. If I was seen there every day they hoped she felt better soon, if I was seen after a gap of a few days, they celebrated our absence in the hospital saying, all must be well. I don't think their job description entailed them to be that nice to patients and families nor did they get any perks for going that extra step, they just did it out of goodness of their hearts.

During the struggle with the disease and treatment I discovered beauty in each day. It was beautiful because my kids expressed their love everyday as they joked with me, pulled my leg and I must share that I do have a foot in the mouth disease. They tell tales of school or my son who is on top of current affairs sagely updates me on them. I love to sing but then I must admit that there is immense room for improvement. I enjoy the looks on their faces when I start with an old Hindi song; funnier still, when they actually hear the original song I have sung and are unable to identify that they are one and the same. I say to them that I was giving the song my own unique melody! The family got together and bought me a whole new set of shoes and bag. In Ditto's words to walk the long corridors of the hospital, I needed good shoes and to carry all the papers I needed that big bag. Lisa was very touched with us finding beauty in random things and commended the woman and the mother I was, while I thought I did need to live up to the standards my husband and kids had set and the least I could do was reflect their outlook. They make me who I am.

There were number of people with whom we had lost touch over the years and they found ways of getting connected again with news of Lavanya's illness reaching them. I heard from Lavanya's Mumbai school's principal and she supported and commended our teamwork calling Lavanya the real hero of the whole story with us being the supporting pillars. I couldn't believe that this learned lady who was the principal when Lavanya was in grade one, now retired, made the effort to find my phone number and E mail. I thanked her for her kind thoughts and words of encouragement, but then I believed that grace and dignity could never go wasted and even from afar it could greatly influence as well as inspire. A fact proven by the number of people, whose lives were touched by her while she was the principal of the school, responsible for laying the foundation of education in our children's lives.

Chapter 13

*"We never know the love of the parent
until we become parents ourselves."*

Henry Ward Beecher

It was almost Mother's Day. I felt sorry that when we were growing up we were not aware of the concept of celebrating the second Sunday in May as Mother's Day. Alas! My mum passed away way too soon. Both my parents are no more, my mum passed away in 1999 due to advanced breast cancer and my dad in 2009 of heart failure. I realize that I didn't wish my mum 'Happy Mother's Day' while I was a child. If I recall right, the first time I would have wished her was the year Lavanya, then all of one year of age walked in with flowers with her dad for me. As I wrote earlier the dad is amazing in showing his love and appreciation for the mum and children are huge learners by observation. Just as I have seen instances in families where the dad ridiculed the mum and the kids followed suit.

Varun buys presents for me through the year, for no reason at all. He probably buys because he thinks of me when he passes through duty free shopping and sees something that reminds him of me, or maybe he sees something that he knows would be appreciated by me sitting on our center table. I realize as I write that I must be the only woman in the world who has never bought jewelry. I might be the only one who doesn't shop for her shoes either. I see that the kids are chip off the block. Ditto went on a school trip to the museum and brought back lovely colorful stones for me. I don't know of any other 11-year-old visiting museum and getting presents back for his mum. Lavanya had bought me an apron and lovely cups when she visited France on a language immersion trip. Both children's artworks adorn our home and I admit I have run short of wall space. Reminds me of the time we were house hunting and went for open houses. Our boy would do a quick walk around and return to inform if there were 'enough' walls or not. I loved watching the realtor's expression.

Anyway, I wished my mother on Mother's Day twice, meaning just for two years before we lost her to cancer, and with my dad I was luckier with twelve years of wishes on Father's Day, until he, too, passed away. Of course they laughed and humored me when I wished them because to them it was weird to be wished Mother's/Father's Day on a specific Sunday of the year when they were parents every day. Should I call them old fashioned or should I say they were realistic? While our girl recovered from cancer, chemo and the works, she baked me goodies on random days. I even received handmade soaps from her, again without any occasion, making me feel doubly treasured. To me, those moments signified 'Mother's Day.' I thought that had my parents been still living, I would have continued to do what I did wherever we were living irrespective of time zone. I called them every day just to say hello, I think that's what made their day as it does mine today, when I receive random tight hugs, big smiles, unexpected presents without occasion and the call out of, "Mummy!" from Ditto as he walks in from school and, "Hey mommy," from Lavanya whenever she enters home.

Many felt that we had a unique family bond. Do I say that the secret of the bond lies in the disease? Well it is true; we had always been a close-knit family but when something like cancer creeps into a loved one, the bond gets stronger with a single-minded focus of letting nothing go wrong. Everything else becomes secondary and you start craving for every small moment together, random meals become special, watching the tele together gains tremendous importance as does sitting and doing precisely nothing in the same room. Varun's job entails a fair amount of travel. When the kids were smaller, to stay connected he would call every night before their bedtime irrespective of his local time. Things have changed now. God bless Steve Jobs yet again, actually rest his soul in peace. Face time is an amazing way to see what everyone is doing, talking to them, even making faces at each other across the globe. Math homework help has become so much easier with us showing him the problem and him offering a quick explanation or E-mail a solution. That I am not a math genius is no more a problem.

I love to watch Lavanya following Varun around the house, trying to run, almost hobbling while he ran ahead of her. He is the giver of 'father of all massages' and she loves to receive them. The moment she would find him sitting somewhere at home, she would sit herself down in front of him, shaking her shoulders and wearing a disarming smile. No words were needed and none expected. Varun would just get to work.

Alpa, a dear friend in Melbourne was convinced that kids are our mirror image and they reflect what we are. I do wonder about that because how does one explain perfectly normal parents having a difficult child. We are born with our unique personality, else how do I explain the difference in the personalities of my two kids with Ditto being an exuberant, happy, excited child while Lavanya is the quiet, happy, inquisitive but not excitable child? The other day I was pleased to find her giggling to herself. Amused, she recounted how Ditto was taking care of her. "He fluffed my pillows, adjusted the cushions and soft toys around me. Asked about the window, checked how much to open, took time to adjust the blinds to that oh so correct angle, put things away, filled water bottle etc. He took time to clear my table, too, again re-adjusting the pillows around me and checking the fan speed." I, the naïve gullible mum, was touched almost to tears at the thoughtfulness of our boy when she burst the bubble saying, "Mommy it was 4.30 p.m.! Homework time for him!" Anything to delay the inevitable! Every time I see the differences between the siblings I am left amazed. While on one hand, she returns home after chemo and if any iota of energy remains in her body tries to catch up on some school work and he on the other hand seems to almost wait for reminders from mum, dad and sister. I never chide him for this, but understand the differences in personalities of two siblings born to the same set of parents.

I was reminded of the time when we lived in Zambia where the society was seeing fewer marriages and more divorces. Step siblings and half siblings were more prevalent than plain old just siblings. Varun's Zambian colleague introduced his sibling to us, very proud, smiling from ear to ear, he beamed, "Meet my brother, same father and same mother!" How unique was that!

Chapter 14

"Everybody can be great...because anybody can serve. You don't have to have a college degree to serve. You don't have to make your subject and verb agree to serve. You only need a heart full of grace. A soul generated by love."
Martin Luther King Jr.

One day we were waiting for blood and platelet transfusion and when the wait exceeded four hours, Lavanya was slipping down on the chair with fatigue. She wondered that food ordered as an inpatient at the hospital took 45 min to an hour to reach her, despite the fact that it needed to be cooked. But blood was comparable to a pack of cereal, coming pre-packaged, requiring no cooking, so why the long wait after a transfusion request! The nurse very kindly explained all about cross matching blood, previous day's transfusion appointment right down to a new requisition during the day, etc. Despite the wait she looked pleased, coloring in one of the little children's coloring books available in the waiting room to pass the time. Gleefully she shared that the coloring bookmakers had become very smart. "When I was little the pages were two sided, color on one side, some activity or more coloring on the other side, but now they make them one-sided so the child can actually cut the page and stick it up without losing the other side." Fascinating indeed!

There were days when a twenty-minute chemo would entail a few hours of wait and both patient and caregiver would return home exhausted. One such evening after a long day at hospital, nausea, pain and evening traffic we reached home to find Varun had starters and mains ready with a lovely bottle of wine chilling for me. He went back to work and Ditto regaled me with stories of the Roman civilization that he was studying in history. I murmured that I really wanted to sleep and he retorted, "Of course, let this be your bedtime story!" So there I was listening to the rise and fall of the Roman Empire as I drifted off to sleep.

We were at a stage of treatment that required weekly lumbar puncture for chemotherapy and I stepped out as I always did as soon Lavanya curled up to get into position. I sat in a nearby corridor and saw a steady traffic of doctors and nurses going in and out of the procedure room. Each one while passing me would say, "She is doing great, she is doing very well," so on and so forth. Three doctors and five pokes later the lumbar puncture for chemo was completed. The nurse was probably as tearful as I was when she stepped out singing all praises for our girl. They all agreed that she was a 'true trooper' and heralded that they hadn't come across any child or adult with her kind of control. As they gathered around a tearful and embarrassed mum, I sought consolation in the fact that their eyes were as wet as mine and that my brave daughter was not in the vicinity to see the scene.

I shouldn't have worried about my teary eyes because I had abundant company right from the nurses, my friendly neighborhood and friends from everywhere. Jayshree laughed to thank God that Lavanya couldn't see all the tearful aunts from Melbourne to Cupertino. I confess I cried again when I read Susan's words from Perth, "Dearest Sohini, this one brought tears to my eyes, God bless Lavanya! You have to be so proud of her! God has a special love for children; he covers them with his protection and always watches over them. Lavanya has so many people praying for her so she will have healing and an amazing tolerance that only God and Lavanya can explain. God bless her every minute and I pray that all her pain is taken away. Sohini, you take care, too. I pray that God gives both Varun and yourself the strength and faith to keep going with a smile! Thank you so much for the updates."

Lavanya was all right, as all right as one can be after five pokes for lumbar puncture. Varun left for London for a two-day work trip and Lavanya got worse with chills/shakes, pain and fever as the evening drew closer. When I called oncology after hours, we were advised to report into the ER immediately. I prepared Ditto to possibly spend the night in a neighbor's home and he went to Srini's home just across from us. Blood works were done and depending on the result another lumbar puncture would follow and by then my brave trooper was crying with abandon. The shivers and chills that set in were scary to watch and I didn't want to think how they felt. One moment her teeth chattered noisily, her body shivered uncontrollably and then she would quieten, to start all over again. She had no control over her body. I felt like holding her tight when those uncontrollable shivers set in but they were far superior to a mum's tight hugs.

Varun landed in London, saw my text and started checking return flight options even before clearing immigration. Our dear precious friend circle comprising of Alka, Usha, Joel, Lubna, Achala, Jayshree, Shilpi, Poonam, Christine, Marion, Alpa, Shruti, both the Priyas, Mona, Aparna, Surbhi, Lisa, Radhika, Ann, all got to work with immediate prayers within themselves and with groups, be it Buddhist chanting or saying Hanuman Chalisa, Maha Mritunjaya path or reading the Bible or the Quran. To those who don't know what 'Hanuman Chalisa' and 'Maha Mritunjaya Paath' are, all I can say that they are scriptures, mantras that are believed to take away all problems, ill health and bestow love, peace, good health, happiness and well-being. We moved to oncology from ER and thus unknown to us then, began one of the most grueling parts of the journey to recovery.

Ditto sent texts to me till about 3.30 a.m. telling all the measures he was trying to get sleep. Starting with counting sheep, going onto pigs, cows, he didn't leave any animal jumping across the fence, to get that elusive sleep. Finally, he too slept. God bless the Srini family for adopting him with open arms for the night. He went to school with their daughter and by the time he returned Varun would be home waiting for him.

What a herculean task for Varun too, flying from California across to the United Kingdom, touch town and return. He was kicking himself for traveling, but then who knew that within 7 hours of his departure fever would set in with chills. He recounted his side of story and that by itself was heartwarming.

At London immigration the officer asked him for the duration of his stay. Varun told him of his changed plan, that he was taking the next flight back home because his child was admitted in hospital. This officer called someone on the phone and another airport employee came by taking Varun aside through a separate exit direct to the suitcase collection carousel. Varun called United Airlines for the earliest return possible and what did the airline do? It arranged for him to fly back by the same flight that had taken him to London. Unbelievable! They arranged everything on the spot, facilitated speedy check-in and within an hour of landing he was back on the flight. I bet all the people involved in facilitating his quick exit through immigration, baggage collection, check-in and immigration again, have this amazing spirit residing within them, to assist just a random passenger, a perfect stranger. Each one went that extra length to help him reach his family at the earliest. I wonder if this book will ever be read in the UK and if they are reading I would like them to know we stay grateful.

My dear husband changed the way he traveled after this incident. He stopped taking check-in baggage. He became a master packer of suitcases, so much so that he could fit his two formal suits with tie and crisp business shirts with a couple of casual wear and shoes into his cabin baggage. No more waiting for suitcases in case of an emergency. By then our neighbors had heard about the latest development. Pat, Pauahi, Srini, Vishnu, Leslie, Gina, Anita, Karen, Isabelle, Greg and Dan assured us that their doors were always open to take Ditto in. Some offered their homes for him to spend the night in case of emergency, while others said they could come and sleep in our home if he wanted a familiar bed and room. There was selfless outpouring of love, help and prayers.

As I write this, I recall that when we were moving from Mumbai to Melbourne my friends and neighbors had joked that I would feel lost without them in the new city. In fact, one of them had said that the only time I might see a face, a familiar face actually would be when I rolled the trash/garbage to the curbside once a week. In India we have this pre-conceived notion that no other country has this unwritten, undocumented open door neighborhood policy where we walked in and out of our neighbors' homes as if they were our own, borrowing that one cup of sugar in an emergency, lending a bunch of cilantro and such healthy expected exchanges. Not that anyone ever took the sugar or cilantro back. I was pleased that I didn't reach Melbourne with any reservations and we were blessed with a beautiful neighborhood and made lifelong friends. When we moved from Australia to America, our Aussie friends were curious, just like our Indian buddies as to how our neighborhood and friends would be in America. They too had this pre-conceived notion that no neighborhood could compare to our Aussie neighborhood, where though it wasn't exactly open door policy similar to India, we were friends and exchanged if not a cup of sugar but, cookies, pasta, salad were welcomed. I was glad to share that we arrived in a neighborhood that was warm, friendly, multi-cultural, with a superb support system through its own google group, which is where I first put up the diagnosis when it happened and the help just poured in.

I realize that if we have no reservation and walk in without those pre-conceived notions, we can embrace a lot more than we would with a closed mind. I am glad we were raised to have open minds and broad thoughts. This helped us to walk into new places with confidence and hope. I was happy to note over the years that our children inculcated the same unknowingly. They can take change in a stride without fuss.

I noted that Lavanya was not herself and I felt something was amiss. She behaved oddly. She was disoriented, seemed lost, scared and cried on and off. It was heart-wrenching to see her big beautiful eyes staring at me blankly and then turning away with sobs. She couldn't understand what I said and was unable to explain what she felt. Help came in the form of the doctor who did her lumbar puncture regularly. She told everyone that our girl was very resilient, so if she was crying with pain it was to be taken very seriously needing high degree of pain management and care. The doctor then turned to her and said, "Lavanya, you shouldn't party so hard that you ache all over." Then she continued, "What no repartee from you! You really must be feeling very bad."

She was put on a drug that eased the pain but made her high. However, the exhaustion eclipsed all other feelings and she lay on the bed without any reaction. The verdict was that the weekly lumbar punctures sometimes caused inflammation around the brain leading to debilitating headache and nausea. I sat in the darkened room praying as I listened to her ragged breathing through high fever. Pauahi and Pat from across the street gave me solace that they had activated prayers for her in their prayer group. The endless prayers continued as we sat vigil by her bed. Alpa, Christine, Priya each sent in full prayer verses. To add to my assurance Shilpi would send me a schedule of prayers that were planned by her friends and her, at different homes around the clock. I thought God was amazing, that he in all his glory made these beautiful souls and put them in our lives. In Lisa's words, "The community of love that you have knitted together, is an amazing force for healing." By the time Varun reached hospital just 24 hours since his departure, Lavanya was on push button hydromorphone. She pressed a button and the requisite dose of the painkiller got delivered through her IV. The frequency of the button being pressed gave the doctors an idea of required adjustments to doses ensuring that there were no possibilities of over dosing.

When I returned home, our 11-year-old boy sat me down and said, "You watch while I clean the house," and proceeded to do exactly that with the broom and dustpan. I did tell him that a couple of days without cleaning sometimes were just fine and we could simply cuddle and sleep. Everyone commended his resilience and adjusting nature to go to a neighbor's home at a moment's notice and also clean the house when he thought mum/dad couldn't. Both the kids showed character strengths that I don't remember possessing when I was their age and I thought of the song from *The Sound of Music*, '*Somewhere in my youth I must have done something good. '* I thanked God yet again for marvelous kids, hubby, friends, family, neighbors and teachers.

Despite her own busy schedule and time difference, Jayshree spoke to me at length from Singapore and Usha constantly WhatsApp'd to keep in touch while Achala stole time in between her patients to give a call to just listen. Sometimes she cried and sometimes she laughed, but between them they held my hand through long dark nights so I wasn't alone listening to my girl's ragged uneven breathing and moans. She seemed to be deteriorating with every passing hour and soon was unable to get up to walk to the bathroom.

With fever touching 40C/104F, pumped with morphine, Ativan etc., Lavanya barely knew that mum had come and dad was leaving. If fever didn't subside there were discussions on a probable CT scan to try to find the cause. Pain was due to frequent lumbar puncture, but the high fever was a concern. Doctors said that during instances like this, the child might take 7-10 days to get over the pain and I couldn't get over this information. I couldn't imagine looking at the shadow of my girl for 7-10 days. Then the nurse compared the headache to childbirth pain and we felt worse. She hadn't moved, eaten, spoken since the time I brought her in three nights ago. While I believed all would be well eventually, this phase of pain and fever was turning out to be very difficult for her to bear and for us to see her bear.

Chapter 15

*"Faith is to believe what you do not see;
the reward of this faith is to see what you believe."*
Saint Augustine.

The frequency of my updates increased in the next few days. I couldn't believe that I was giving updates as regularly as I was. I so desperately wanted everyone to join in with prayers because by then Lavanya was completely disoriented. She couldn't figure out anything. She was unable to hold a glass of water to take her pills, with no comprehension of which hand held the glass and which held the pills. If we tried to help her with medication she got irritated and in turn confused with the irritation.

In view of the unexplained fever and all other complications, the chemo scheduled for the next day was cancelled and she was taken for lumbar puncture to check the spinal fluid for infection. At the procedure room she had a seizure and was immediately moved to the Pediatric Intensive Care Unit (PICU) – her second visit since diagnosis two months back.

With goosebumps all over me, I sat at home with Ditto, reading Varun's text that a CT scan was on, to be followed by lumbar puncture. My poor baby, so very brave all this while, was bawling her heart out. She couldn't understand what was going on or why. I too, then wondered why! We had been positive and continued to be of the final result of complete cure, but this phase was daunting and so unfair on a child and her family. I implored to all to pray and pray hard, for my normal girl to be back soon with those oh so honest opinions, acute observations and that subtle sense of humor.

I had been having a spate of monologue in my mind. All through I had been a huge believer and had strong faith that when God gets you to it, he sees you through it. Since Lavanya's first diagnosis in July 2003 my prayers, acts and thoughts of prayers had increased immensely. I didn't impose my thoughts and beliefs on anyone, as religion and prayer are personal choices but I began fasting on certain days, for both my children's health. Call me superstitious but I gave up eating particular food on particular days. Funnily, I took care of entire prayers department for the family. I even commended myself for not losing my faith with a second diagnosis on March 26th 2013. In fact, it just strengthened my thoughts and beliefs, and I worked harder to feel good with prayers combined with positive thinking. I read books on healing; I heard and played mantras to have positive energy flowing through our home and mind. I didn't preach much but I practiced a lot, however, suddenly

I felt this tsunami of emotions shaking my un-shakable belief in God Almighty. I told Varun, while also sharing with Achala and Jayshree that I had a good mind to vacate my home of all things related to prayers- our numerous idols of Ganesha, some acquired by us during our travels and many others gifted by family and friends during their pilgrimages. I was raised in a home that had a separate room for the Gods. Yes, the idols even had their own little beds, pillows, side pillows, mosquito net, beautiful clothes and ornaments and were adorned with fresh flowers every day.

I was shaken to the core with Lavanya's latest side effects, that affected my strong faith. Varun's quiet patient listening probably helped because I don't think that I would have been a good listener at that moment. Achala, too, heard me out all the way across the oceans in Melbourne, again quietly, while Jayshree scolded me gently. After much lamenting to them and fighting countless silent battles with God I felt the beginning of healing to regain that momentary loss of vision. I was in the process of regaining my faith because that was what was living for me; I realized I couldn't live without my faith.

With Lavanya showing no signs of life except for the monitors showing her breath, heart rate, blood pressure and pulse, our phones buzzed with WhatsApp, viber and sms from all over. I compared this to the first time she was sick in India in 2003 when I didn't have this support group or any other. Varun and I were each other's support group with a few of our friends from his office and old/new neighborhood. Now that we had worldwide prayers on twenty-four hours, I sat back with hope in my heart and prayers on my mind. My belief was fighting its way back into me and I welcomed it with open mind. My crisis updates had our world coming together to provide support in the only way it strongly believed- prayers. Lisa said that she had never prayed as much as she was praying then and I think it was true for most.

Ditto yet again warmed my heart and soul when he showed maturity beyond his years by saying, "It would be better if you send me off to someone's home for some time, then both of you could be with Lavanya in the hospital without worrying about me." Was our boy really 11?

Varun updated me about the 'Code Blue' emergency call given at the time of Lavanya's seizure. It was strange as well as scary when one heard a code blue/code red on the hospital speakers but it was alarming with huge degrees of fear when it was given for your child. He heard sounds of running from every direction. He was impressed to see an immediate arrival of doctors, nurses, cardiologist, anesthetist, ICU specialist, oncologists, chaplain, security, Lavanya's social worker Kate, the doctor who did her lumbar puncture and the list went on. She was stabilized and moved to the pediatric ICU.

Varun, too, was treated with utmost care and attention. The Chaplain assured him that they were all praying and Kate stuck along with him until things settled down, just in case he needed something. An IV line was put up in no time on her elusive veins. The port already had an array of tubes connected to it. She had black and blue marks all over her arms and legs later, that showed how many people had tried to find a good vein.

When awake, Lavanya continued to be disoriented, having severe anxiety attacks, losing control on everything. She lay there without speech, movement or recognition. She was a blank face with a scared soul and we continued clueless. All chemotherapy was rescheduled till the situation was solved. It is at times like this one questioned one's faith, one's belief and trust and came back a full circle to continue with the same hope that there had to be a light at the end of the tunnel. I kept wandering in this vicious circle, hoping, praying, questioning followed with more hopes, prayers and questions. There were no pauses, commas or full stops. Ditto corrected me by saying that in America apparently it is 'period' and not 'full stop.'

En-route to the cafeteria to get lunch for Varun and me, I would meet doctors, nurses and others who had treated Lavanya sometime or the other in the last two months and each had something to say. I commend their memory because despite seeing so many patients everyday they remembered her name, her problem, her latest situation and had something nice to contribute, something positive always giving me that support. I said so to one doctor who was on rounds on week two of her treatment and he replied, "Of course I remember her, she is a remarkable girl," and I bet they said that for each of their patients because these children were indeed special. I prayed that the MRI and CT scan took place without issue or anxiety attacks as each time someone touched her she would go into a full blown panic attack screaming, shivering and losing control. Everyone said that this would also pass; I hoped it would be today rather than tomorrow. My neighbor across the street, Gary wrote, "My work place has a chapel and I will stop by before going home to pray. I will do this daily for you and your family until she comes home. Stay strong!!"

We spent our days with her, talking to her despite no reaction, recognition, response or movement. We sat around her and chatted about daily mundane things attempting to create as much normalcy as possible. I believed that she could hear us in some profound subconscious depth of her mind and know her loved ones were with her. Shilpi had sent me many texts and I could feel her angst while she fretted over our girl's condition, so helpless to do anything from so far except pray. I wrote to her that it would appear strange coming from me, but since I practiced it I had to tell her. I realize that for a caregiver, parent or anyone closely connected to the day-to-day activities in the life of someone going through something like our girl, could be very overwhelming. To give our best, to judge rationally, to make the right decisions and have a conducive atmosphere around is extremely essential. To achieve this, I felt it was required that one must stay slightly disconnected otherwise everything overwhelms what should/must be done on a day-to-day basis. The focus might change making things much more complicated. Everyone deals with difficulties in different ways and I found this working for me. As a parent, or a loved one it's very easy to feel the pain but that pain makes one emotional taking the focus of caring away. I could be wrong in my thinking, but I didn't know of anything else that could work better. I felt talking of happy times or normal things helped immensely and I believed it was not escapism.

A friend from Mumbai requested access for her cousin to our blog. She felt that he might be uplifted with the story of a teenager against the disease, her battered body rising after every fall and her mind fighting the heart wrenching side effects. I was proud to be the mum of children so special, each equipped with amazing grace that cannot be taught. I knew that not only were our friends learning from the children but so were we. One doesn't learn only from the educated, trained, grown up and experienced persons, one can learn from children too, and life's lessons at that, which are far bigger than any math, science or language art.

It would be an understatement to say that it was an eventful night. Lavanya's BP dipped to 70/33 and more intervention began, with more IV meds and new monitors being hooked up. Auto BP measurement every 15 min irritated her but couldn't be helped. With all the action happening post-midnight I was without my contact lenses or glasses and every time the BP monitor buzzed I would walk up to the monitor to see if the BP had stabilized. Yes, every fifteen minutes I walked up to the monitor and turned back to my little place on the sofa at the foot of her bed. The nurse from her station outside monitored the same but she did look confused as to what I was up to with my regular short walks. She laughed with relief when I told her the reason, else am sure she would have thought that she had not one but two confused patients in her care. With all the monitors beeping, BP machine making its own music, Lavanya suddenly called out – "Ditto, volume!! Lower the volume." I was delighted to hear her complain, say anything at all and further elated that she realized that he wasn't around as she asked, "Where is he?" Everyone around smiled and agreed that it was indeed a good sign.

Ditto – I know the world is a beautiful place with wonderful people and the same is being proved time and again. Ashwin called to say that his family and a few others were going to Lake Tahoe and wished to take Ditto along. We really didn't want Ditto to feel that he offered us just a day back that we could send him somewhere and we were jumping at his offer. Varun asked him and he was delighted with happiness. Ashwin's children and he were of the same age. So we would see my little rock, so full of wisdom after four days. Just the other day when he saw me with tears, he said, "Think of all the good times we have had, look at her old lovely pictures and feel happy."

Finally, all the test results came in and it was confirmed that the seizure had been caused as a reaction to spinal chemo. We were to continue in the ICU until she stabilized. She was onto her fifth day without food or drink, though getting slightly oriented and having better control of her body. The worldwide virtual vigil continued.

Chapter 16

After almost a week I had good news – Lavanya's BP had stabilized from those scary lows to 93/55 levels. Her pulse, too, had come down to 100-110 ranges from 120+ range. Mail brought the awards that she received from the Grand Concourse for French that her teacher Ms. Finck very kindly and thoughtfully sent with a note. I brought them to the hospital to cheer her up but she couldn't read due to blurred vision. So yours truly read French to her and after days of lying blank, crying in pain, Lavanya giggled and smiled. Clearly my French reading, accent and pronunciation needed divine intervention.

Another improvement was that she appeared more lucid. She was stable enough to realize that she was hallucinating on and off. Suddenly she told Varun, "Daddy, why are you playing the flute!" Then giggled, "And why would daddy play a flute?" She thought she was in her friend Aditi's room in Mumbai, with pictures of clouds on the ceiling but a semblance of reality made her think she was in the 'day hospital' which had twinkling stars on the ceiling. Then suddenly she asked, "Oh why did they change the music from nach baliye (Bollywood) to Beethoven?" The only music in the PICU was that of multiple monitors, doctors and nurses monitoring her. At one point she saw Disney princesses coming out of the glove boxes on the wall and smiled happily looking at the wall. The boxes were labeled as per hand size, S, M and L and she saw fairies and princesses including Tinker bell emerging from those boxes. Though to us, seeing her eyes happily follow imaginary figures emerging from the glove boxes was frightening. Next she leaned over to see how the game was proceeding since she thought that we were in a bowling alley and looked confused when she didn't find any alley, balls or pins. The doctors laughed that the ICU with all beeps, monitors, doctors and nurses did resemble a party place. Later we laughed over it, but when it was all happening it scared the living daylights out of us!

Usha was bowled over that in hallucinations our girl could see fairies as she had heard people saw demons, bugs and nothing nice. She was amazed that the hallucinations, too, seemed to be fun and positive. The night nurse while leaving said, "I will be back tomorrow night and if you are still partying in the ICU, I will take care of you." I knew our girl was on her way back when she whispered a thank you. Priya from Delaware rejoiced in delight feeling that we could all take a breather and Shilpi followed up with continuous prayers. I realized that we weren't the only ones with our breath suspended in continuous prayers but our world was with us. One night in a semi-conscious state she said – "Daddy, can you fix me?" He quietly but emphatically replied, "YES."

When Lavanya read my updates she remarked, "Hey, mommy, surely you made all that up!" Varun and I smiled yes, just to liven up the blog we added some spice but we were very happy that she had no recollection of her loony times. I say an innocent mind is a brilliant mind when one day our boy came up with a brilliant idea. He wanted to know more about leukemia and I sat him down and explained all that I knew. It surprised him that Lavanya had to undergo this grueling treatment that made her sicker than better. Why not take blood from all of us and change her full blood! While I knew all would be well it still rankled me and I shared Varun's explanation to me to strengthen my belief. In his understanding her entire system, that's hematology, was being 'rebooted.' It was being done in every possible way, 'shut down' with every medicine known, systematically to 'restart' afresh. So with every chemo her counts dropped, sometimes to almost zero and then started building up again so eventually they would all work well as they were supposed to. It was a team effort between the WBC, platelets and hemoglobin and their Mother Port the bone marrow. Somehow this explanation seemed to make sense to all, right from Ditto in Cupertino to Shilpi in Singapore.

Lavanya received her first reiki session from Namrata while she was still in a semi-conscious state in the PICU and thereby began our journey with reiki to last us forever. Lisa, the chiropractor was thrilled that reiki had begun as she felt that was perfect for Lavanya. Simran, just two years Lavanya's senior sounded very mature when she wrote that her classmate had learnt reiki for about two years and according to her it really does help to mitigate pains. The positive energy flowing through the body acting on the hormones coupled with the faith might help her feel better.

One morning, one of the oncologists on rounds asked Lavanya, "So, hon, tell me is the neurologist taking good care of you?" While Lavanya quietly nodded the lady further explained that he was her husband, so Lavanya should tell her if she needed anything. She joked, "We at oncology take care of everything so we can teach neurology some." What a huge contrast from ten years ago in Mumbai when Varun's colleague Deepak and I had gone to meet a renowned oncologist in an equally renowned cancer hospital for a second opinion. He was too busy to see another child or another parent for a second opinion despite an appointment. We had waited until he finished clinic and he came out with his subordinates in tow to glance at our reports with apparent disgust that we wanted a second opinion. His expression said it all and his words confirmed, "Why do you want a second opinion? It is all written here. I have nothing to add!" I had felt as if he had punched me. Varun's colleague looked equally shocked at the callous way we were spoken to. To add insult to injury the doctor accompanying him smirked to ask, "You do have another child, don't you? Why do you worry then?" Needless to say, I was blown away by these uncouth monsters who were supposed to be healers. I quietly walked out as fast as

I could, as far away as I could get from those cold unfeeling men, also known as doctors in that renowned cancer hospital. They, of course charged huge fees for that walking consultation in the corridor, but I had no regrets. On the contrary I was brimming with happiness that we were not in their care. I would never see them again and our girl wasn't anywhere near them. I am convinced there are none like them because our treatment in Mumbai was smooth with the best of doctors in medicines and bedside manners. In Stanford, if I asked the doctors ten questions, they would answer patiently, if our girl asked twenty more, they still answered patiently, sometimes shaking their head and at times laughing- "Girl you are a hard one."

Though the hard one by then had developed a reaction to all pain meds, with morphine giving hallucinations and the others inducing nausea. The ICU team thought that ibuprofen might help but the onco team was against that as it contradicted with the treatment protocol. Nine days of no movement had them putting vibrating bands around her calves to help the blood vessels get some exercise. I must say I quite liked this kind of exercising. They sounded like someone's gentle snoring. I had to smile to myself as I warned the night nurse to expect some sound show as Varun stayed the night with her – reverberating snore at her head where he sat and gentle small ones at the foot with the regular BP machine and all other monitor sounds.

As if there wasn't enough going on, next she developed pancreatitis, again another chemo medicine induced issue that would go away on its own. That though made her slightly happier because it entailed no eating and drinking. There were efforts beginning to get her to eat and drink something, but with this new issue, attempts at eating and drinking came to a stop. She got new bags hanging on her IV pole, one was TPN (Total Parenteral Nutrition), another had in all upper case letters written in bold- **FAT**!! We were told that TPN was calculated specific to patient requirement of energy, protein, minerals and other nutrient necessary. All pain meds were stopped due to reaction and she was sedated until she felt better. It was kind of boring with her wisecracks, comments and observations missing.

As her hallucinations had more or less gone, fever, too, broken, we were moved to oncology after a week in the ICU. Amongst the doctors, nurses and specialists who responded when 'she coded' (hospital term for an emergency, code blue sounded across the hospital) one was an ICU specialist, Dr Mahapatra – a person of Indian origin, raised in Thailand and for the last decade or more an American. He laughed as he told us that everyone said Lu vaanya coded and as they got her vital signs etc., and kept calling out Lu vaanya and he kept correcting them, "How will she respond if you are not calling her by her right name – say La van ya." We smiled that she answered to both, as many said her name with a short 'u' after the 'L' rather than the long 'a' and anyway, what's in a name? It didn't change who she was and how brave she was being. In fact, in times of extreme endearment I call both my kids and husband things I like to eat. It can be the name of a vegetable or fruit or even a dessert and guess what, they all respond and I would probably never understand how they figured out which one of them am calling out to.

With what's in a name, I am reminded of the time when we lived in Kuala Lumpur. Initially when Varun and I would walk into a party, many of our local friends would look towards us and say, 'so many balloons.' The first few times I looked behind me expecting to see plenty balloons but as time passed we realized that I was Somany and Varun was Balloon.

Our friends showered us with virtual medals and certificates on parenting, humor and resilience. Reading all the lovely words I could almost feel the glow of halo around my head, see the cloud beneath my feet and then I came back to earth because I knew that anyone would do what we were doing. Any dad/mum would take care of their ailing child the way we were; there was nothing extra-ordinary about what we were doing. Extra ordinary was how the patient, our girl was handling things and the sibling, our boy had risen up to the occasion. Extra ordinary were the people surrounding us. Varun and I were mere parents doing what any parent would do.

Chapter 17

"Our life is the creation of our mind."

Buddha.

The receptionists from the day hospital joked that Lu vaanya must love the hospital since her stay in oncology continued. The pancreatitis seemed to have fallen in love with our girl, refusing to leave, showing an upward trend. All scheduled chemo was canceled until that settled down, pain reduced and counts recovered. The oncology team sent the pain management team and we learned many more adjectives to describe pain – acute, shooting, crippling, sharp, dull, throbbing, burning, chronic, pinching, cutting, nagging, etc.

Namrata came by with reiki for Lu vaanya, dinner and a marvelous book for the mum. The book called the *Biology of Belief*, by Bruce Lipton discussed that our cells may be controlled by our thoughts. Now all I had to do was read it and get the naughty cells in her body to behave. Contemplatively, that's what we had been unconsciously doing. We had driven the leukemia cells out, raised her counts and armed with the proof in the form of a book we could only strengthen those beliefs. Lisa was very glad to know that the next chemo was being put off and that we were getting acupressure beads and treatment. According to her acupressure and reiki were very good non-invasive approaches to pain and nausea. There are many books written on image and thought-based approach to recovery. There is also an excellent program developed by Jon-Kabat Zinn on Mindfulness Meditation that incorporates very gentle yoga. She suggested we could read the entire thing in his book *Full Catastrophe Living*. Each chapter gave a simple meditative exercise to try each day and a very simple yoga move. She went a step ahead and gifted me the book on kindle so I could read at leisure. God does really take care in adversity because I couldn't find an explanation as to how we carried on day-to-day normal life; get up in the morning, bathe, pray, cook, eat, drive to hospital to our girl and then one of us went back home on time for our boy to monitor homework – sit with him, cook dinner, eat and sleep to repeat the same again and again, day after day.

Lavanya came out of sedation to chat with me for the first time in almost ten days from the day we drove into ER. I brought her up to date with all that happened while she was sleeping. She cried that she wanted to go home, like yesterday. We imagined us sneaking past everyone, giggling at the sight we would present. Lavanya hobbling in her ridiculous hospital gown dragging the IV pole with multiple monitors, bags and tubes and me in my bright yellow dress would be conspicuous.

One night she whispered, "Daddy, you hold my hand while I sleep," so daddy dear held her hand. When he thought she was deep asleep he gently removed his hand, only for her to clutch at it again and say, "I will make space here for you to sleep next to me holding my hand." I don't know for how long Varun stood holding her hand. Knowing him I knew he could do that for eternity.

The books I had been reading made me talk to her about the power of the mind. I said, "Tell your lipase to go down, your WBC, platelets and hemoglobin to come up, talk to your counts, talk to your body, instruct it to behave," and she giggled, "Food come here!!" Lavanya next asked the doctor if it was okay to chew the food and spit it out. After two weeks of fasting her hunger and taste buds were craving to munch on something. He laughed but had to say no as that, too, would agitate the pancreas. Lisa suggested that everyone try creativity by drawing shrinking lipase, increasing WBC, color them with crayons; also use play dough to make these seemingly silly things fun and fruitful. She even drew how the cells are supposed to look. We were impressed, warmed and humored as we imagined lipase and WBC being drawn in different parts of the world. I bet they had not been looked at artistically until then.

The counts decided to behave finally and showed an upward swing so she was taken off two IV antibiotics proving that the WBC and platelets not only heard us but also listened to us. She was allowed saltines with clear broth. She compared it to something no one should know, and it did look awful and unappetizing. We thought that maybe the chicken broth was not great as Lavanya could barely drink it, so veg broth was ordered. Both were hot water of different colors though Lavanya begged to differ. She went into more detailed distinguishing factors that I would let people's imaginations work on. However, it was an improvement from sips of water and crunching ice chips.

Just when Lavanya was preparing to suggest to the doctor that he should try the chicken and veg broth before recommending them, he said he would let her eat a low fat diet. Highly excited we phoned the dietician and she said sorry, she couldn't send low fat diet as the computer told her Lavanya was still on a broth diet. What a letdown! However, after much excitement of tracking down the doctor to change the order on computer, a meal of Asian wok comprising of brown rice, snow peas and carrots were ordered. Oh, to see her happily crunching the snow peas and savoring the brown rice was a picture I would treasure for a long time. It was more than two weeks since her last meal. Shilpi was all smiles as she visualized our girl savoring the snow peas, crunching them happily and Lisa danced all the way to her kitchen to make her special Pumpkin Love soup.

A team of six doctors visited Lavanya to share the good news that they were planning to improve her diet and work towards getting her fitter for a discharge after resuming chemo. A dietician visited to plan and discuss the diet with her. And then it all came crashing down as she looked solemnly at our girl with very sad eyes to whisper, "Lu vaanya, you are having a hard time and it is only going to get harder. It is bad and it will get worse." I saw my husband's face changing and my girl's big eyes getting bigger. I understand one has to do their job that may at times involve being the bearer of bad news, but surely that news, too, could be coated and said in a way to not make it sound worse. I would say it's an art to give bad news so the person receiving it doesn't feel miserable.

So the rude mum had to step in. I told the dietician that if she could keep to the specifics of the dos and the don'ts we would be grateful. She didn't really have to get into detailed description of the situation. We could decide how good or bad the situation could get ourselves without help. Mind it, I wasn't rude, in fact I smiled and said with all due respect. Probably she was taken aback but she tried to keep on course. Thereafter, every time she would get into superlative adjectives like terrible, difficult, tough, bad, worse, she would fleetingly look at me and change her sentence murmuring something like, "Oh but probably you can manage that." I am sure she meant well, but she was the first bundle of negativity we encountered in this happy sunshine place. As soon as she left, Varun gave Lavanya a big long hug and she just held on to him. Moral of the story was that she was allowed 5 grams of fat per meal, not exceeding 15 grams a day, no more than 400 calories in twenty-four hours.

Lavanya's Chemistry teacher Mia Onodera visited and Varun forewarned me that the next time I drove to hospital, I needed to carry extra handkerchiefs and lots of tissues. The teacher had left a handmade quilt and cards. A quilt made of school colors of purple and white with numerous patches from both students and teachers stitched together to make the most unique quilt ever. The quilt carried messages on each patch from Lavanya's teachers and friends at Monta Vista High School. Her friend Yana had drawn a beautiful picture of *The Lion King* and written Hakuna Matata, which literally translated means no worries, or don't worry, be happy. The English teacher Frank Ruskus had been very innovative and had drawn the themes of the books they were reading that year in class. Dad and daughter were convinced that mum was going to get tearful on seeing it. Well, guilty as charged! Just the thought of it made me teary eyed. How could one convey the gamut of emotions that overwhelmed us, our gratitude in their thoughtfulness and our appreciation for their kindness? There were no appropriate words. I did wonder if I walked around with a constantly overwhelmed expression or not! One of the quotes I truly believe in is, "Where there is great love, there are always miracles."

Chapter 18

"There are far, far better things ahead
than any we leave behind."

C. S. Lewis.

It was almost time for schools to re-open after the summer holidays and Lavanya was busy convincing her oncologists as to how good she felt and how she was an ideal candidate for discharge immediately. I was very surprised when they said they would consider the possibility, but everything was dependent on her counts. By then we had given genders to all medications, saline and heparin calling them Mr. Methotrexate, Mr. Cytarabine, Ms. Heparin and so on. Counts were Mr. Count but someone commented that it sounded like Dracula, so we made Count a female, and we all waited to know how Ms. Count was doing.

Then one day I received a mail that I had to share with all without disclosing the name of the writer. One would expect a woman of probably my age or so to generally have clear thoughts and sensitivity, but when a 15-year-old shows that remarkable degree of maturity, understanding and compassion it is an unusual combination; it just bowls one over.

"Hello Sohini,

On behalf of all Lavanya's friends, I want to say that we congratulate her with the end of her sophomore year and her first year in America. We all wish her strength, love, and a big happy miracle. We all kiss her and hug her, and want to say that we hope a good summer will begin for us all.

Lavanya's friends and I understand that Lavanya is going through a very hard time and does not have much time for visitors. But if she wishes to see all of us at once or in small groups, we want to say that we all want to pay her a visit at home or in the hospital if she feels well or has a wish to see us. Her friends are always there and she can count on them.

With love."

Written by her friend, all of 15 just like her and new to the country just like her. As I said I was completely bowled over, though Lavanya didn't seem surprised and actually expected nothing less from her friend. Lisa felt that gratitude, positivity and hope were always reflected back as it was doing so for us. This young girl went ahead and made a roster for visitors complying with Lavanya's treatment schedule with no visitors on the day or soon after chemo.

With an upward trend in Ms. Count the much-awaited discharge took place and viber, WhatsApp, Facebook messages worked overtime over the globe as messages of congratulations poured in. Someone wrote, "I am opening a bottle of my treasured precious wine today to celebrate." Varun and I too shared a wine and watched silently as our kids slept in their respective rooms looking like angels. Honestly that's a sight that always moves me! Whatever the kids had been up to during the day, pranks included, they all looked like angels while sleeping, and not just my kids but all children around the world.

The next morning for our hospital visit, I asked Lavanya if she wished for a scarf or cap and she said, "Oh it's just the hospital. Everyone is more or less like me, balding, so no need. Actually I could go to school, too, without it if it's as hot." I looked up to my girl for being unselfconscious and confident against all odds. Ditto returned from school very excited and intrigued with all he learned in ancient civilizations in social studies. He animatedly told me about all that he found interesting, similarities and differences with today. He was most intrigued with reincarnation, rebirth and the soul living on. His exact words, "If one is born again and again, I would like to be born to you in all my births." Speechless for a moment I recovered fast enough to give him a big tight hug saying I would love that, too. Then he thought some more and said, "But that's not possible, because you will get old and your soul will leave your body. So you could be born to me and I to you and we could keep borning to each

133

other!!!" I know, I know that there is no word called 'borning' but whoa! I thanked God again and any surprise that I was moved to tears! Indeed, I would just love to be 'borning to each other.' Just when I get that nagging doubt, hoping that he was not feeling neglected with all that was going on, he would reinforce my faith that somewhere in my youth I really must have done something good.

I used the days that I didn't need to go to hospital and Lavanya didn't need much attention to write thank you notes to everyone. It gave me a warm pleasure to express my family's appreciation of everyone. But the one person I couldn't convince that we were managing fine was my sister. Every time I spoke to my sister she would feel terrible about her inability to be with us, as she herself was not keeping good health. Likewise, for my brother-in-law who, amidst all odds with my sister's poor health, had also assured of his presence next to us, with just that one call. They had been with us during Lavanya's first episode of leukemia. My ever caring sister kept wishing that she could be with us and even suggested that she could come and stay at home thereby having someone for Ditto all the time. However, her own health was giving her so many issues that we couldn't have her travel the long distance.

Chapter 19

"Volunteers do not necessarily have the time,
they just have the heart."
Elizabeth Andrew.

The more I met our oncologist Dr. Lacayo, the more highly I thought of him. As we waited almost an hour for him in clinic, Lavanya passed time pointing out things and wondering what they were. She couldn't figure out a phone that had receivers on both sides but only one keypad, and on enquiry we found that it was the interpreter phone. She wheeled herself around the tiny room on the doctor's little stool instead of sitting on the patient examining bed. Just as she was having her 'wheeee moment' of sliding across the little room on the doctor's stool, in walked her oncologist and gave her a big amused smile. Just as she started getting off her perch he said, "Honey, you look comfortable there, so carry on," and happily sat on the examining bed. What an easygoing man! He knew that she was well enough and old enough to not fall off the stool. After examining her and generally chatting about her school, junior year/grade 11, subjects, how she would manage, he turned to me and asked, "And how are you and your husband doing?" That was so sweet and thoughtful. I had never heard this from a doctor before, asking the parent/caregiver about them.

He wished to know more about the days when she was knocked out and hallucinating. He asked her if she saw bugs or crawly, creepy creatures around her. He was most keen to know all the details of Barbie Disney princess coming out of the doctor's examining glove boxes. A nurse walked in and congratulated her on her French award and Lavanya drew a blank saying which French award. We reminded her of the award she received while she was in the Intensive Care Unit. She had no recollection! On returning home I showed her the certificate, medal and Madame Finck's lovely letter in French, reminding her how she had laughed when I had read it to her. She drew a complete blank from that week. An MRI was repeated and it was noticed that the trauma to the brain was almost gone but that week was a blank hole in her mind, probably forever.

In the hospital there is this gentleman, anywhere between 80-100 years of age, who is one of the many volunteers involved in cheering the children with stories and presents, his way of giving back to the place which cured his son some three decades back and now the son is a father of two children. I felt very touched when he said, "When I see you smiling, I feel very happy, I have to send something for Lavanya for the happiness I get," saying this he gave me a necklace for her. Even though she was not an in-patient he still thought about her, he didn't really need to send anything except his wishes and prayers but he thought a 15-year-old might appreciate a necklace, simple plastic silver beads and of course she loved it. Christine, an optometrist and professor in Melbourne University, Australia, wrote, "Sohini, volunteers are such precious assets to the hospital environment. They are often touched by adversity in their own lives and somewhere in the mix they too, become touched with a love and generosity only born from such experiences. They continue to touch others struggling and so on and so forth. Wish this was a routine observation but alas!"

We, too, hoped to volunteer at the hospital one day. Lavanya visualizes us waltzing through the corridors with her telling the kids that hey, just a few years back I was where you are, so hang in there! I couldn't quite see myself as 70 plus distributing pens and necklaces to mums and kids like the happy elderly gentleman but yes, I hope to give back to this institution that is curing our girl and giving her a new life. The gentleman I write about, the volunteer, he is an epitome of dignity as he carries his son's and grandchildren's pictures in his wallet or shirt pocket. He would always tell me, "If she gives you a bad time don't think about it, it's not her, it's the medicines." And I would assure him that she had been co-operation personified. I couldn't have wished for a better child. Lisa wondered, "How is it that we all derive encouragement and positivity from one who is living through such a difficult ordeal?" I agreed with her as I looked at my family and derived endless strength. I soaked in their positivity, absorbed their love and I didn't need anything else. My husband is a special rare kind of a man. His little gestures make me feel loved and cherished even though he doesn't pour the love out verbally. The other day he wished to cook us fish and returned from the grocery store with the fish all right, but along with that he brought yours truly beautiful flowers. I could just melt in all that unspoken love.

I went to school to get the junior year summer reading books and met Mr. Hicks, the assistant principal. A gentleman who we hold in very high esteem, again assured me that it was NOT important for Lavanya to read them through the summer even though they would have tests as soon as school began. It was NOT important for her to attend school on day one; if she could, then well and good else whenever she was ready they would welcome her. Her teachers wrote to her that all she needed to do was concentrate on getting well over the summer while, here she was planning her first day back at school on day one after holidays. The co-operation and understanding of the school surpassed every expectation leaving us astounded at the kind of support possible and provided in a public school of a small town.

Mary Jane, from Melbourne said that she realized that the simple things in life become ever so precious. She felt that it was also blatantly obvious as to how much she had taken for granted and it was time to reflect on this on a daily basis. She added that she prayed also for the bright days and times that I described to continue and for them to be the norm rather than the exception.

During our visits to the hospital, some days were routine, some days would have some hiccups and then there were days that would stay with me for a long time due to something unusual or special. On one such visit, as we continued our wait in the pediatric oncology, an apprehensive looking lady, approached Lavanya and asked her, "Do you like your port?" A surprised Lavanya replied, "Yes, it's okay." The lady asked further, "Does it pain? How was it compared to the PICC line?" Then she elaborated that her son was to get the port the next day, he had the PICC line at that time. Lavanya, too, had graduated from a PICC in the arm to a port so we could understand where she was coming from. I felt so proud of our girl when she explained to the lady at length, concluding with, "Port is better than the PICC." On knowing that her son was just 4 years old, Lavanya further assured her that, "It is less painful for smaller kids than big ones like me so he will be fine." The mother almost had tears of relief in her eyes as she thanked her profusely for explaining all details. I was happy that Lavanya could put her mind to rest. I didn't have to imagine what the lady was going through, I knew it.

The next time we visited Stanford for chemo we had a wait of two hours plus, though we saw much and learned lots during the wait period. A grandma walked in with her probably five-year-old granddaughter for chemo and with them came the most well-groomed, well dressed, calm and saintly dog, a therapy dog that the child needed to cuddle every time her port was accessed. I hadn't seen a better-behaved child/adult than this dog. No restlessness or panting, no huffing or puffing, barking or sniffing anyone. He came in and sat like a perfect gentleman next to her stroller. Then he went in with her for therapy and we saw him again on our way out sitting at the back of her stroller in a little bag. We came away very impressed with his trainer and him. I had to call him a saint because of his gentle eyes and calm demeanor. Little did we know that soon Lavanya who was scared of dogs would be cuddling and petting therapy dogs that visited the Bass Center for childhood cancer while waiting for chemo.

As we walked into the short-term chemo room for therapies under 30 minutes we saw the nurses and some administration officials entering the room with a cake, candles and balloons. They were celebrating the 'Happy End of Therapy' for another patient, probably a 6-year-old and there were celebrations all around. The curtains of all the cubicles were drawn so everyone could join in and other patients and mums, too, clapped and sang. Volunteers gathered around clapping and adding to the rejoicing, making the occasion memorable. How lovely was that! Shilpi teared up on reading about the six-year-old's end of therapy celebration and thought that amidst the transition and glitches, the celebration by the hospital team was indeed heartwarming. I too agreed that they went that extra step to make things simpler and special for us patients and families. Lavanya decided that for her end of therapy celebration in the hospital she would bake a cake, for herself as well as for all the staff we saw day to day. While the six-year-old didn't appear to understand the importance or the novelty of the occasion I could see the tears in her parent's, family's eyes and there were no dry eyes amongst the adults, in a room full of patients' mums, dads and families.

As we drove back Lavanya said that she wanted to celebrate. Puzzled, I asked celebrate what, and she said, "Celebrate that child's end of therapy." Well I wouldn't mind celebrating a perfect stranger's therapy conclusion either. It did feel good that someone was done with the treatment. Since her counts were not too low to be in a public place I phoned Varun to check if he and Ditto were free. We picked up our boys and went for an impromptu pizza party near home. The four of us dining out for the first time together in months and the great occasion was celebrated in a big way.

Varun was to travel to India thereafter and as we packed we heard Ditto talking constantly. On peeping in we found him reading a history chapter to her as she listened with rapt attention. I was delighted with the affection and helpfulness between the siblings until Lavanya burst the bubble with, "I promised him a chocolate if he read me a chapter!"

Chapter 20

"I can enjoy anywhere, and I can leave it.
Life is about moving on."

Waris Dirie

Varun was to go for another work tour and going by history had returned every time, as Lavanya had become a guest at the hospital. For that particular trip, after Varun's departure both the kids decided to join mum at night to sleep. So yours truly had the pleasure of being sandwiched between the two with all their paraphernalia. Lavanya with her water bottle, (yeah, she takes it to bed and keeps it next to her pillow, not even on the bedside table), kindle and Ditto with his little buddy, the most cuddlable elephant. Every time someone turned the bottle would go bang on the floor or Ditto's elephant's tail would tickle my nose or the quilt would be pulled on one side. After much tossing, turning, adjusting, grumbles and complains by all, Lavanya decided to go back to her room as she missed her army of pillows and cushions. Last I counted she had six pillows, four cushions, a big fat panda, a cute though big lion and I wondered how she slept between them!

Anita, my neighbor came by with a bag full of plums from her tree. There was so much that we would be making everything, entrée, starters, mains and desserts with plums for a while which reminds me that it took us some time to get used to certain terms in the States. While entrée in Australia meant the starter, in the States it's the mains! The funniest was fresh off the boat, we wondered about the TOGO signs in many restaurants here. While we thought it was a strangely named chain restaurant, it turned out to be the Aussie and Indian 'take-away,' actually means 'to go' and not TOGO. Just like initially when I would ask someone where I could throw the trash and get blank looks followed by an excuse me! What is trash to Australia is garbage to America. I might have adapted to many American ways of life from the Aussie and Indian ways, but one thing that even after two years plus bothers me is the indicator of American made cars, blinking red and not amber when turning. We grew up seeing a vehicle change lanes with a blinking amber light indicator but in American vehicles the same is a red blinking indicator confusing me between brake lights, taillights and indicator lights. Then there is another light! A traffic signal is called the traffic light. Someone giving me directions once said, and you turn right at the light. I was like, what? Which light? If asking for directions in India, you would be shown the direction with the hand pointing to a direction, with instruction, go straight, turn right at the tall brown building, left after the fruit vendor, right again after passing a huge tree. Sometimes those passing by too would join to add their inputs. In the States usually it went something like, go north, turn east after half a mile, turn right at the light, but I say the Japanese take the cake in giving directions. Reason being, they never give directions; they would drop you to your destination. They would either walk you or get in your car or take you in theirs. I am talking of the Japan I lived in, more than a decade back and things may have changed now but I do have fond memories from then, of the times when strangers walked me to my destination. Yes, I admit I often got lost while exploring with my children, one in stroller and the holding on to me. Steve Jobs and Steve Wozniak were yet to get together to provide us with GPS or map on a phone.

We have been married for twenty-two years in which we have moved twelve times, lived in eight countries covering four continents. It's the miracle of love that we survived and thrived amidst all the changes and it's the miracle of our children's personalities that they adapted to all the changes by indulging in Skype talk with friends in Australia with an Aussie accent, only to change to an Indian accent when talking to buddies in Mumbai and of course the American English locally. I can vouch for the miracle of technology that we are still connected with people we met in the countries we lived in. While I carry fond memories of all the places we have lived in, each one stands out for something extraordinary. When Lavanya was diagnosed the first time, we had recently left Japan and our Japanese friends got together to hand make a thousand origami cranes stringed together to bring good luck to the leukemia patient as per their folklore. It's been over a decade but the cranes have also moved with us, occupying a place of honor in every room Lavanya has occupied since she was a little girl of five.

We reached a stage of treatment where Stanford arranged for home labs for Lavanya and we progressed to a stage of weekly labs from almost daily labs. By then home schooling, too, had settled in with two teachers from the district coming home two to three times a week to help her catch up with school work and we were falling into a new schedule with lesser hospital visits.

During the next blood transfusion, Lavanya developed chills and that was the end of transfusion and beginning of another long stay at the onco ward with me trying to figure out a place to leave Ditto until Varun's return. That was when I realized the power of the blog. Gita and Namrata within moments of my post on the blog got in touch with me to take Ditto with them. Ditto was soon packing his bag to go and stay with Namrata who lives in the same neighborhood as us. We were hopeful of a discharge in 48 hours. The ever thoughtful Namrata was even getting him later to see us and deliver my overnighter, which I had transferred home to get the car cleaned, else the hospital overnighter was a permanent fixture in the boot. Lisa, too, soon followed up with, "Do you need for me to come spend the night at the house with Ditto? I will finish with patients around 6:30 pm. I can also drive up there and pick him up and deliver him to someone's house, or I can stay with Lavanya for a few hours while you take Ditto somewhere and get things for your overnight if that is what you need to do." With each passing experience my gratitude and amazement at the people power, love of the people in our circle kept multiplying.

So we were at the hospital, hooked and booked with Lavanya sedated and blood transfusion resumed. I was chatting with Usha (God bless WhatsApp), and I told her that I had phoned Ditto once I knew about the required stay in the hospital. I advised what to pack for his visit and stay at Namrata's home and all he asked was for how many days did he need to pack and what was going on. There were no whines or complains, nothing! Just an unquestioning acceptance, a co-operation beyond expectation or hope, which actually made me kind of sad, happy and scared all at once.

She put my mind at rest by saying, "We think we teach our children about the world, when actually they teach us. That acceptance, that fortitude, that ability to internalize all conflict that Ditto had demonstrated – it's what scriptures say. Kids are born with it; we make them lose it along the way." Lisa's view was that Ditto was learning that his family was far bigger than he realized and it was a wonderful new aspect for him. She was pretty confident that we couldn't have 'untaught' him anything but he was learning all about grace, gratitude, generosity of spirit, faith, hope and love from us and all those around. It was only natural he responded and behaved the way he did. Wise words from her for I saw many siblings in the hospital who were not exactly the fortitude of love and patience as they waited for their sick brother/sister to receive treatment. I was feeling a terrible conflict until then as one of us was always there with each child at the end of the day but then when I saw him completely at ease with Namrata and looking forward to a pizza dinner I knew all was good.

Lavanya meanwhile was quite bored so she answered all the questions on her white board. Each room had a white board with colorful markers which gave the doctor and nurse in the shift, details from previous shift, what the patient wanted to do, needed to do, family time, parent's contact number, etc. Things like 'what I need to do today, where is my family focus time, my queries, were printed on the board. Usually Varun and I wrote our questions and concerns there with the permanent marker provided. Sometimes we made a note there that we had gone for a quick coffee if she was asleep so the doctor/nurses knew where we were and that we were returning soon. Anyway, Lavanya filled it up with, 'family time as scheduled at home today, when am I going home and I want to go home now.' In addition, she drew faces to pass the time, all with deadly comical expressions!

I realized that we were not going home anytime soon and I was going to miss Ditto's robotics events. When I told him that, for the first time I heard a tremor in his voice that made me feel terrible. This was the first ever event that neither parent would attend, else we made it a point to be present, one of us at least in however small or big an event. I consoled myself by saying that there would be many more.

As expected the lab works showed that we didn't make the counts! The ANC (Absolute Neutrophil Count) needed to be 500 for a discharge and our girl was at 350 the next morning. As I said before, ANC or the Absolute Neutrophil Count is calculated as a percentage of total WBC with neutrophils and the normal range is between 1500-8000. The 24-hour blood culture was negative and the long wait for the next labs began.

Namrata brought Ditto along and something really special for me. She went and video recorded his robotics presentation. The children made things with Lego and got them to move, syncing with computer. I was touched beyond words at her very thoughtful gesture. Malini couldn't thank Namrata enough for adopting Ditto and was amazed at her thoughtfulness of recording the event for me. I admit I was tearful later as I thought about her kindness. What an amazing soul! While she stayed with Lavanya, I went home, showered changed and returned. Low ANC didn't allow anyone to share Lavanya's bathroom so either I could bathe in the public bath outside or go home, and I preferred the latter as it was just 15-20 minutes' drive away. With the day drawing to an end, the sun going down I started my prayer for Ms. Count.

I have said often enough that the world has been shrinking and distances becoming negligible with virtual distances at zero. Joel called and Lavanya complained of boredom so he told her jokes and riddles, long distance from Mumbai. She wished to see Mumbai rains, auto rickshaw, traffic, noise and those were shown, too, all thanks to face time on I pad!

Every morning we waited for 10.00 a.m. to know if Lavanya's counts showed an upward trend and each time we were disappointed as it continued spiraling downwards until it touched rock bottom at ZERO. So with nothing other than to wait we joined the hospital organized entertainment for the day. That particular day Disney Pixar animators were invited to draw for the children affected by cancer and the new movie *Monster University* was screened on the TV of each room. So this lovely young gentleman came in to draw for our girl and offered to draw anything from Disney. She wanted *The Lion King* and he sheepishly said, well that's really old. I draw the new ones, all monsters, goblins as shown in the new Disney movies. Disney is no more about cute little things but furry scary things. However, he very kindly obliged and attempted and drew a lovely picture from *The Lion King*. The next day some football stars were expected and Lavanya was asked whose autograph she wanted and she was ignorant, "I don't know anything about football." While she was explained as to how famous those people were, I smiled thinking of the reaction of the boys down the corridor. Again I was amazed at the ideas the hospital presented regularly to keep their patients entertained. Achala's son on the other end of the world at once wished to know the names of the players who were gracing the patients that day and I thought America or Australia, boys will be boys!

Chapter 21

"The aim of art is to represent not the outward appearance
of things, but their inward significance."

Aristotle

I always told my kids that one could learn under all circumstances, from any age, at any age and anywhere. It was proved right yet again when Gita visited with her lovely trio, Ananya, Ananth and Anuj aged 12, 9 and 4. Lavanya was all smiles for the entire four hours they spent with us despite their packed schedule. The kids were amazing, with no awkwardness about her hooked up to monitors, her scanty locks, her mask, the loud beeps of the monitors or the periodic vital checks. They took a short walk to the gift shop amidst giggles, feeling very responsible as to who got to push her IV pole. Gita bought them all almond joys and it didn't feel like a hospital visit and I told Gita, that they miraculously made a long boring

150

day short and sweet. Ananya with her mum's help made an elaborate blanket for Lavanya in her favorite colors of green and blue. Our girl was getting enveloped in blankets of love and each one will be treasured.

I thought of the morose looking family sitting in the lounge of the onco ward and their equally sad looking visitors and thanked God for the party times, joy and fun our visitors brought us. The child life therapy personnel dropped by to check if our girl needed something while Gita and kids were visiting. He looked genuinely pleased with the exuberance in the room and wondered if the kids down the corridor could also join. Truly our friends were special; they touched not only us but also others around us.

As I did Lavanya's scanty locks, I joked what hairstyle would madam like, a ponytail, a pigtail or a bun? She came back with, "Mum make a French braid!" There's this old Indian joke that we often laugh over, a woman having three strands of hair went to a hairdresser and asked for a beautiful hairstyle. The hairdresser said, "Let me braid your hair for you," but as she was braiding her hair, one strand broke so she said, "Oh, let me make a bun for you," but then the second strand, too, broke and the hairdresser was left in her oops moment. The understanding lady shook her head with one remaining strand to say, never mind, "I will leave them open, free flowing." I too did exactly that with our girl's hair.

One night as we slept, the door of Lavanya's room opened at 2.00 a.m. and her nurse came in with the charge nurse. I was told that we needed to move. Lavanya needed to be shifted to cardio as an emergency/serious case had arrived and needed a single isolated room. As Lavanya was the 'most stable' on the onco floor she was chosen for the transfer to cardio into a sharing room. My girl asked if she was stable why couldn't she be discharged and share a house with her family. Well, the answer was that she still needed the IV antibiotics. So while stable was good news, it was ironical that she wasn't stable enough for a discharge, just a shift to the 3rd floor to cardio as oncology was full.

Cardio floor followed a protocol of attaching patients to all gizmos and monitors but Lavanya told them she was not attached to any of those in onco and so was left alone. The kid across the curtain needed her light on and Lavanya is someone who sleeps in a pitch-dark room. It was past three a.m. and we were sitting at one of the cardio lounges, as she was unable to sleep in the room. She passed the night reading *The Kite Runner* while all I wanted to do was sleep. I tried to read the book I carried but instead stared at the dark night through the glass wall of the corridor. My phone lit up with a message from Varun that he had landed in New York and was taking the next flight to San Francisco. I saw the morning dawn with the first ray of light in the sky as we sat in the lounge and prayed that the day brought good news about Ms. Count. The nurse got her morning blood draw and antibiotic ready. The sleep deprivation suddenly didn't mean anything as I realized that the child across the curtain was a hematology–cardio patient with Down syndrome.

When I shared the latest on the blog, her being the 'most stable patient' was greeted with great cheer and relief. In Lisa's words, "I have a crazy idea; maybe we could all simultaneously pray for or visualize Lavanya's

ANC jumping up at a set time. I guess we devotees are spread across the world so that could be tough to time. Another fun idea could be for us all to draw pictures of Lavanya's neutrophils rising and reproducing and take photos and post! I will start!" I too, had read about visual imagery being helpful. I didn't really know how WBC or ANC looked but I was hoping they increased. She in turn said, "There are tons of books and support groups in the Bay Area that teach visualization and meditation for healing. Dr. Bernie Siegel started the whole trend and he has many books. This is NOT a new technique and is highly researched." She also added that her mother suffered from breast cancer for seventeen years and visualization helped her in many ways. I thought of my mother who had suffered from breast cancer just like Lisa's mother, though didn't survive beyond five years from diagnosis.

In India in the 1990s, no one around us knew about visual imagery and my mother didn't receive the benefits of alternative therapies like these. At that time alternative therapy was family combined with home remedies. In Christine's words, "The concept of visual imagery being used to initiate change is not new and has been gaining momentum in neuroscience and neurodevelopmental literature." Lisa went a step further and sent pictures of how neutrophils looked and started drawing them. Needless to add, our friends got to work too with their pens, pencils, crayons and markers. Namrata and Surbhi told me to visualize a glow entering Lavanya's body. Lisa recommended that we think about the neutrophil increasing so there I was ending the day with thoughts of healthy glowing neutrophil all through our girl's body. The visualization increased by leaps and bounds, artwork of neutrophils multiplying kept us laughing as many of our friends sent in their version of neutrophil and WBC. With due apologies to all the budding artists some of the neutrophils were hilarious. We received drawings of neutrophils with big smiles, jumping neutrophils, glowing neutrophils, fluorescent neutrophils, neutrophils doing the Spiderman jump, neutrophil in superman suit and neutrophil had turned into a superhero. The WBCs looked like Casper the friendly ghost.

Everyone wondered how to visualize the hemoglobin increasing and I was reminded of one of my first manicures in Mumbai, a few decades ago. The lady in the salon had accidently drawn blood while cutting my cuticles and then had the audacity to say, "My, my, your blood is so dark red, which blood group?" I had almost shrunk back expecting fangs jutting out any moment! So thinking of this I told my friends that probably we could just imagine dark red blood coursing through her veins.

Lisa took visualization to newer heights when she bought a bunch of blow bubbles in bottles, the kind where you unscrew the cap and dip the circular bubble blower into the solution and blow bubbles. The bubbles were visualizations of Lavanya's neutrophils and she was passing them to everyone she met in the next few days and everyone she knew would make neutrophils for Lavanya. She had them in her clinic and all those consulting her blew bubbles for Lavanya's counts as they waited/came/went. The corner was called, 'blowing bubbles for the lady' and of course the neutrophil drawing would have given Pablo Picasso a complex. In Shilpi's words, "Am a huuuuge fan of our bubbles lady and the bubbles corner in her clinic had me stunned, blown over would be the right word actually, totally awesome."

The art and the artists kept us motivated and full of hope and it dawned on me that many of our artists were doctors or worked in the medical field. We had a rare combination of panel of experts right there on our blog, from GP, gynecologist, pediatrician, dentist, optometrist, chiropractor and orthopedician.

It occurred to me that when one normally was accepting, without complains and was generally appreciative, it did make a difference. The night we moved into the cardiac unit, Lavanya spent it in the lounge outside the unit due to (in her words) live *Grey's Anatomy* going on in her shared room. I made a noise, a tiny bit of a noise, that maybe before she was allotted that particular room mate who needed critical care intervention requiring a dozen of doctors and nurses in the room, probably a small amount of research could have helped her to share a room with someone who was as stable as her, not requiring a team in and out of the room through the night. Nothing against shared rooms but sleep was important when one's platelets were 19000, hemoglobin was 7 and WBC was around 500.

Just a fortnight back I had sent a letter of appreciation of the services we thought were great, a positive feedback. This time, I was contemplating on a stinker when action happened. One of her oncologists worked things out at the cardiac floor and Lavanya was moved to the quieter part of the cardiac unit away from all the action, beeps, busy nurses and crying babies. It was mentioned that since we were 'usually co-operative parents' they tried to accommodate us in a quieter part of the unit though till today I wonder as to why the word 'usually' was used.

Chapter 22

"When you are a nurse, you know that every day you will touch a life or a life will touch yours."

Unknown

I was amazed at the number of tiny babies needing heart transplants, valve replacement and other heart related surgeries. When Lavanya said her back ached, they gravely informed her, sorry we don't do backs, only hearts. The cardiac unit looked like a day care with little red buggies being driven around by the nurses with the baby contently cooing into the nurse's phones as other nurses cooed back from across the room doing the mommy talk. Surprisingly there were few mums and dads staying on the floor and I assumed they must have been going to work and returning late. Most amusing and sweet was when I saw a non-Spanish-speaking nurse trying to be a Spanish-speaking mum and saying hola hola from across the corridor into her cell phone that she had used to call another nurse who held it to this one-year-old boy who wanted his mum. He showed his beautiful toothless grin thinking his mum was on the phone. Then I saw this man probably in his 40s as a patient in the pediatric cardiac unit and was told he had a congenital heart problem that was fixed at birth by the very same unit. He was there for a routine checkup and review. Since pediatric cardiology had fixed him, he needed to go back to them for consult and review. We thought that the adult patient amongst all the kids was kind of cute.

After days, we finally had an upward swing of counts from 0 to 3. Well, it wasn't a leap but it was the first time since admitting that the neutrophils had gone up. We had a good night's rest in the single room in the quieter part of the cardiac unit. Lavanya was thrilled that her day nurse, a Fijian Indian's name was Usha, one of her best friend's mum's name. Small things could bring much joy, just like every time I went home I would give Ditto all the coffee change I had remaining in the pouch. Last I gave him was 18 cents and he was over the moon! I, too, learned to find much joy in small things, like 0 to 3 gave us joy, I learned to look at the bigger picture.

The good news was that her platelets had recovered on their own without another transfusion. Funny bit was that the auto-correct kept making the 'their' in the above sentence to 'her.' I guess the platelets were also to be called Ms. from then on. The platelets actually didn't go up, 'they' jumped; I somehow couldn't bring myself to calling platelets as a she and say, she jumped. They jumped from 19000 to 84000. For her next chemo, the first day of 'interim Maintenance 1' she needed an ANC of 750 and platelets of 75000. Well at least she had made the platelets, ANC would also come up with everyone working hard in all corners of the world, though the world is actually a sphere, without corners. Just to protest against all the weird depictions of themselves the neutrophils might just jump very high.

Our girl was delighted when her French teacher Ms. Finck visited and Varun told me that she had been on a high the whole day thereafter. Namrata added spark to the day by getting her soup, crackers and chips in addition to reiki. I returned home that afternoon to spend the much-needed time with Ditto. Mother and son had a date, *Monster University*, Japanese dinner and cheesecake dessert. Gosh! One should have seen his expression of glee and happiness, he was just short of jumping, actually he jumped! Though I love to watch kiddy movies, I prefer the animations of the olden days. Did I just call my childhood 'olden days?' I like the fairy tale story line of the old Disney movies with prince, princess, kingdoms and palaces as compared to the furry fury fights that are so popular now.

When a port stays accessed for a week, meaning the needle stays on the port giving IV nutrition, chemo drugs on and off through seven days, the needle needs to be changed at the end of the seven days to avoid infection. Hence Lavanya needed to be de-accessed and be re-accessed again and she decided it was going to be one with an audience. The other day when Joel made his daily call to speak to her she asked him as to why he never wrote anything on the blog, never a comment or anything. His take of, "But I talk to you every day!" didn't help and she said she would like a few words on the blog from him. Ah talk about demanding women! The man obliged and here goes what he wrote, "Irrespective of the counts being low, Vander's spirits are always high. And in those high spirits she insisted that it would be re-access time with a difference. This time I would HAVE TO (no choice given) watch her on Facetime getting re-accessed. I wouldn't volunteer watching someone getting an injection; I look the other away even when I get normal blood works. However, I grudgingly obliged after fussing a bit, considering this was one of her less demanding requests. (The more demanding requests in the past have been make my pain go away, get me all A grades). Luckily for Vander and me the re-access was performed efficiently. Vander, of course, made it all appear very painless and easy. Now we are waiting for the counts to do their part." Vander is the name given to our girl by Ajay when she was all three years of age following him and Joel around when we lived in Tokyo. They used to sing, "You are my vanderwall (Wonderwall by Oasis)," and she would run to them. She is seventeen now and she remains Vander to them while Ditto is called Detox.

After enjoying the hospitality of the cardiac unit for a few days we were back at onco floor getting a warm welcome by the familiar nurses, surroundings, kitchen, etc. Even the white board in her room had 'Welcome Back Lavanya,' with a smiley face that truly brought big smiles. We had accumulated quite a lot of bags, board games over the weeks stay so we piled Lavanya's bed high with everything while Lavanya and I walked with the transfer and charge nurses down to onco floor. The charge nurse of the stem cell unit took over at the entrance, wheeling the bed ahead of us and we overheard, "Hey where is the patient!" The patient was following behind beaming and even did a little jig in the privacy of her room. The warmth of the nurses in the onco floor was both touching and a remedy for speedier recovery.

Onco floor saw a jump in Ms. Count from 3 to 4 while the platelets leaped to 114000. I wrote to our friends on the blog to help create history by praying hard to make that never seen before jump in the counts. Maybe it would be written about in research books eventually, how group prayer and visualization for a certain child brought up ANC from 4 to 400 in 24 hours. I met one of the mums who had been guests on and off at the onco floor with us and felt a little fearful of what was in store for us, because she shared that it was their fourth week of stay for exactly the same reason as ours – waiting for Ms. Count! I felt a shudder go through me at the thought. Otherwise, Lavanya was doing fine and Ditto was waiting for 19 July when he would fly off to Lubna and Nafis in New Jersey for ten days. Our drama king had a big calendar in his room, and crossed out dates with exaggerated precision every morning showing the final countdown to flight, checking out suitcases at home, various sizes and shapes of toiletry bags and the list was never ending. Whatever he did, he made us smile.

Amidst all the stories of counts I had to share something funny – the onco floor is a 'no touch floor.' Meaning everything is automatic using sensors, the toilet flush, the basin, the soap and the towel dispenser. No touch meant no transfer of germs. Immense and repeated importance was laid on hand wash as that was what stopped the spread of infections. I realized that one gets accustomed to things very quickly as I would wait with my hand under the basin tap for the water to flow or under the soap dispenser for the soap to be dispensed and feel quite foolish when realization would dawn that I wasn't in the onco ward of the hospital. Call me silly but the sticky mats at the entrance of the onco floor would often have me in splits. There were these huge sticky mats on the floor at the entrance of oncology, and the moment someone entered, the dirt from their shoe would get stuck on the mat. But very often I would see the shoe, too, stuck behind and the person hobbling ahead only to turn back either laughing or self-conscious to retrieve it. I, too, am guilty of losing my shoe to the mat a few times only to run back giggling to retrieve it.

After more than ten days, the labs showed that counts had jumped to 60. Lavanya and I had a bet the previous night whereby she had said that it would crawl up to ten while I said it would jump up to a hundred with us deciding that anything above 50 would be my win! I do love these kinds of wins. I have to write Shilpi's words as they came, "Dhinka chika dhinka chika dhinka chika dhinka chika hey hey hey hey hey hey." Christine wrote that she was at a vision neuroscience conference at Melbourne University and would get all her colleagues to start visualizing as well. I got goose bumps as I thought of all the optometrists in an Australian conference visualizing for their colleague's Indian friend's daughter in the United States. Macarena wrote in, "Just so you know we are visiting Barcelona and in every church we visit a candle is being lit for Lavanya and her counts, there are many churches so many prayers from us, too." And I thought hey neutrophil; you don't stand a chance!

Seeing the cultural, racial, educational and continental diversity of people of all ages wishing and praying for us I was reminded of something I had read that made a lot of sense to me. It talked about the 'third culture kid.' It's that kid who was a little confused with the question, "Where are you from? Or where was home?" For this kid home was not a place, but the people in it. This kid has had amazing sensitivity training – real life – and would take off footwear in a Chinese/Indian/Japanese household while not showing soles of shoes in an Arab home. They celebrated Christmas with the same gusto as they did Diwali and enjoyed biriyani on Eid or went trick or treating during Thanksgiving. This kid felt incredibly lucky to have loved ones and memories scattered all over the globe and knew that McDonalds tasted drastically different from country to country.

I was happy that I could say that our children were the third culture kid. They were not confined to a place, culture or mindset. A friend wondered the other day as to where all the people on our blog were from, our friends, our supporters and our prayer group. Last I looked we had Melbourne, Perth, Sydney, Singapore, Kuala Lumpur, Mumbai, Delhi, Pune, Nagpur, Kolkata, Dubai, Abu Dhabi, Bahrain, Turkey, Sweden, London, Hamburg, Cologne, Italy, Pakistan, Russia, Delaware, Oregon, New Jersey, Minnesota, Connecticut, California, Mexico. I probably missed some but yeah all in all we had it all covered here – our own United Nations, culturally, racially, religiously as diverse as could be. I have said before and I truly believe

163

that if the Gods of all religion got together for tea they would find the prayer for a certain teen a common constant.

We were surprised when one day Lavanya's nurse told her that we made the nurses feel good. Apparently we were the only family in all of onco that addressed each nurse by her name and not just 'nurse' or 'excuse me.' While I am surprised that no one else addressed them by their names I am glad this little attention to detail made them feel good. They worked so hard and we noticed that most of them worked at being nurses with a passion and not addressed it as a mere job. I realized that the reason they were exceptional at their job was because they didn't consider it a job. No wonder we tell our children to follow their passion, expertise and success would follow.

It was the 4th of July and Varun with Ditto arrived early in the morning with breakfast and then went to P.F. Chang in Stanford Shopping Center next door to get lunch. Just as we finished the nurse came and whispered that there might be good news of a probable discharge. The ANC had shown a strong upward swing too, as charted by Lavanya on one of the white boards of her room. It was truly Independence Day dawning.

We really didn't want to anticipate and plan so we just took it easy and lo behold, the doctor arrived and said, "All counts are on an upward swing, no fever, no chills, nothing grown on blood or urine culture and since we were a good responsible family he would let us go." Whew! I don't know how I controlled the jig I wanted to do as he spoke. I told him that I was resisting the urge to hug him. It was fun to watch this new young doctor turning red with embarrassment. He was yet to encounter and get accustomed to a parent's joy and exuberance. I did believe that the ANC and platelets, the recovery had shown an upward trend all because of the prayers of our friends. Their prayers, wishes, lighting candles, visiting temples/churches/chapels/mosques, reiki and more, collectively achieved a miracle in half the expected time.

Chapter 23

Lavanya's primary oncologist with the nurse practitioner gave the thumbs up for proceeding with the next stage of treatment. We were to begin high dose methotrexate on the 11th July 2013 and were also told that the treatment would end exactly two years from the start of this phase. So 11th July 2015 would be the last chemo, signifying the end of the treatment. I realized our daughter would be a double graduate then, High School graduate along with Chemo graduate.

In this stage of treatment called the Interim Maintenance 1 lasting 56 days we would be hospitalized every two weeks with a small twist to the story. The medicine would be given by way of IV for 24 hours and then to flush the drug out it could take any number of days from 3 days to 14 days. Day 1 and day 29 of the protocol would entail a lumbar puncture with chemotherapy. The spinal chemo was to take place in the Stanford branch of LPCH (Lucile Packard Children's Hospital) while the remaining chemo was scheduled at another branch closer to our home at El Camino Hospital at Mountain View. So after the spinal chemo our girl would be wheeled into an ambulance and be driven to the other branch. The doctor joked that if she wanted more excitement they could have the sirens on, but of course there were no sirens as we were not in a life-threatening emergency. We thought if Ditto were allowed into the ride he would talk about the incident probably for years. As the spinal chemo also involved bone marrow tests for MRD she would be under the effects of anesthesia and not be really aware of the transfer to the other hospital. Her friends and she found it hilarious that she would get an ambulance ride. I still don't understand the teen sense of humor. What is funny in an ambulance ride under anesthesia!

Our last experience with spinal chemo had been difficult, causing brain inflammation with debilitating headache, backache and seizure requiring an ICU stay followed by three weeks of hospitalization. She again asked the doctor as to how often her treatment would allow her to attend school once it started after summer. He in turn asked her when her SATs were and suggested that four days prior to SAT he would stop her chemotherapy to avoid chemo fog in the brain, another known and routinely felt side effect.

Jeremy Clarkson, Richard Hammond and James May provided her with much entertainment and she couldn't get over the fact that millions including her dad and brother watched *Top Gear* globally to 'just hear about and see cars.' If she had her way she would walk or bike everywhere. Machines just made her sick! Phew! And to think she wanted to start driving lessons! God help the instructor and the dad. Not too long ago she showed great interest in what I was doing when I drove while she sat behind. The conversation went something like this, "Hey mommy what are you doing?" My answer was that I was pressing the accelerator. Next came, "And now what are you doing?" My answer was "I am still keeping the accelerator pressed." "Okay, and now?" Well, the answer didn't change. Then came a very indignant, "What do you mean? You keep your foot on the accelerator all the time? You can't press it once and take your foot off, fold it under you and sit comfortably? You mean you can't sit like the auto drivers of Mumbai? What if I wanted to scratch my toe? What if I felt something inside my shoe? If there are two pedals, one for brake and one for accelerator why do you use only the right foot for both? Why not one with each foot?" And I thought again, God save her driving instructor!

Between our amusement on the probable driving lessons and 24 hours long chemo, Radhika phoned from Mumbai to say that someone wanted to talk to me. That someone turned out to be the house help/maid/lady Friday who worked in our home while we lived in Mumbai. In India, one has the convenience of having household help every day, as much as one wants for whatever work one wants. It could be one or multiple persons, depending on personal preference. They could be hired to cook, clean, iron clothes, do your hair, babysit your child, etc., you name it, you paid for it and you got it. So we, too, had this lady who came to clean the house and do odds and ends for a few hours every day. Now Radhika's lady Friday saw a few tears on Radhika and knowing the reason was Lavanya's health promptly went and told my lady Friday from yesteryears. It's a small world out there and everyone knows everyone else. So my lady Friday landed up in Radhika's home to speak to me. This uneducated lady with a rich baritone of a voice, a richer heart, who worked in our home, all of the five and a half years that we were in Mumbai assured me that all will be well, Lavanya will be fine. My thoughts went back to the time Lavanya had leukemia in Mumbai, the very same lady held my hand as we cut away blotches of hair that kept falling on her food and cleaned up with me every time she threw up. I yet again realize that high education, culture/social/economic structure were not what made a person memorable, but it was the thoughts, words, actions that made one remarkable and cherished.

Then one day I received a call from someone I met while we lived in Zambia in 1996, someone who became a great friend over the years – Prema. She phoned to say that she was coming to Pennsylvania and Chicago to drop her two kids (The same two kids I babysat in Zambia when they were both less than four years old) at college and if it was okay with us she would like to detour and come to California to see Lavanya. Okay? No, we were not okay, we were delighted and looked forward to that visit.

169

Varun's engineering days buddy, Hari, phoned to say that he and his wife Surekha were planning to take Ditto to Connecticut for the rest of the holidays, teach him guitar, piano, skate, swim, whatever to keep him happy and busy through the holiday. Suddenly the summer holidays seemed too short to do all that our dear friends wished to do for or with our boy to keep him occupied. Achala from Melbourne said that she wished and hoped to see all our friends someday as each of their personalities had touched her in some way. Usha hesitantly asked me if I felt that she was stalking me as she sent messages with assurance of prayers every morning and evening. I welcomed these stalking messages, as they were all prayers and blessings for our girl to recover fast, with minimum issues. It made us yet again realize the power of the human mind and kindness of the heart. Alpa wrote beautiful words that were very humbling, generally pointing out the fact that positive vibes produced positive action bringing about all round spirituality, happiness and peace.

To numb the port site prior to access we would apply a numbing cream, lidocaine. At one such instance as we sat in the lab and the nurse got ready with the paraphernalia of blood draw, beginning with wiping off the cream, spreading the sterile napkin to keep everything, Lavanya told me to turn around. At home we have had this naughty game of giving a playful little poke, nudge, push on the back to one another while passing by. I wondered if she was inviting me to turn around in public for that little poke/shove; surely she didn't wish to give me a fun poke like Asterix and Obelix, in the nurse's presence. While I did comply by turning, both the nurse and I enquired why. I was tearful when I heard, "I don't like to get poked, but mum likes it even lesser, so it is better if she doesn't see." One day she hopes to get these pokes without the mum in the room. Varun jokes that by the time her treatment is done she would in all probabilities be brave enough to access herself while standing in front of the mirror if allowed. Meanwhile I wondered what was worse – to see your child's port getting accessed with a one-inch needle or just hear that little sigh she let out when the needle went in.

During the transfer from recovery room to the ambulance, the ambulance staff going through her records suddenly exclaimed, "Ah I knew I had seen the dad! I knew it! I knew it!" It so turned out that they, too, had responded to Lavanya's code blue so suddenly there was a familiarity born out of shared crisis. Varun left the recovery room earlier than us, as he needed to retrieve the car from the basement parking and Lavanya held his hand whispering, "Where are you going?" On hearing his reply that he would follow the ambulance in the car she smiled, "Come, come, we will have fun there."

While Lavanya slept with the twenty-four-hour IV chemo on, I went through our blog to update and realized that most of the regular commenters had developed a rapport and respect for one another without actually knowing or having met each other. Something only beautiful selfless people were capable of doing – liking, admiring, appreciating and respecting without meeting. They all held our hands, gave us strength with their support and prayer and we knew the great things that had done for us. They had formed a chain of love, engulfing us in a kind of confidence that could be imbibed only by love. That sunny day in July 2013, I requested them to add in their prayers a very dear friend who had been diagnosed with breast cancer. I didn't disclose her name until she reached that level of acceptance and comfort to share her diagnosis and treatment but Mali turned out to be a brave heart and braver soul. She combated breast cancer head on with strength, dignity and grace.

Achala felt that there were so many emotions flooding through her, thinking of Lavanya anticipating fun in a new hospital and encouraging daddy to join her in the fun despite all that was on. Truly, laughter with friends and family was the best tonic was her verdict. She assured us of prayers for Mali too. Lisa coined the names – Lavanya the leukemia destroyer, while Mali was the breast cancer destroyer.

By then our blog readers had become a very focused learned group. Everyone wished to know what specifics to visualize next. The high dose methotrexate was known to cause havoc from mouth sores right down to the esophagus, nausea, vomiting, headache and drowsiness. Patients were known to find eating, drinking, swallowing, talking difficult and so I thought forearmed with those facts everyone could direct their energies to heal all above. The hospitalization after the end of the 24 hours IV was to monitor the kidneys, as that was an organ feared to suffer major side effects. I had to smile when messages of thanks poured in. Our friends were thanking us for letting them know what to visualize. They amazed us, touched as and humbled us every day with their thoughtfulness. Susan said that she sent love for both, our girl and our friend and that she had already started praying for her, too. It was great when people prayed and interceded for us, took the pressure off and in the Bible it is mentioned that pain gave one remarkable strength. In the words of Mary Jane, "We are praying for minimal side effects and pain for Lavanya. We are praying, too, for your friend whom we all know of, through this site. All will be well for both. Sounds like a worldwide joint hug is needed for all who are privy to this site.

"Sohini, I hope I'm not stepping over the mark here, but personally, I would like to say a huge '*thank you*' to all your amazing family, friends, teachers and all others who have been 'hands-on' and given, and continue to give help and support to Lavanya, you, Varun and Ditto, in a multiple of ways. Being across the world, I have been unable, due to distance, to physically be of help, but wanted to thank those who have. These special people are so worthy of all your praises. Their want to help is a reflection of the incredible, caring and giving family that you are. I give through the power of thought and prayer and will always do so."

When I read Mary Jane wished to thank everyone hoping she wasn't stepping over the mark by doing so, I thought gratefulness had no mark or limit and if one was thanking people one hadn't met for doing good to another that was a unique personality trait one displayed. I had heard somewhere that love couldn't be divided, it could only be multiplied.

Chapter 24

It felt like a beautiful day had dawned as the sun seemed shining just right, the coffee perfect, a re-energized Lavanya after sedated sleep was strong enough to walk with a more normal posture as compared to her hunched over after Bone Marrow Test and lumbar puncture. Varun and Ditto arrived to spend the whole day in the hospital. In fact, it all looked very good with the drug level in the blood showing it was moving out, urine tests showing kidneys remained unaffected.

It was always intriguing to find nurses and doctors turning up with interesting conversation, sense of humor and something to contribute in our ongoing conversation in the room. Like the time Varun was massaging our girl's shoulder, the nurse who came in at that moment paused to exclaim, "Oh that looks awesome! Dad my turn!" I always commended them in my mind and in words whenever I could, that, "Ladies, you are doing a marvelous job."

The highlight of that day was the fund-raising event by ACS – The American Cancer Society, that held an annual relay run to raise funds, awareness for cancer as well as to honor those fighting the disease and in memory of loved ones lost to the disease. Karen, another lovely neighbor had hosted a luminary in honor of Lavanya in the relay that was a beautiful event held in Cupertino High School Grounds. Varun and Ditto attended it where the names of all those in whose honor luminaries were donated were called out and prayers were offered. Lavanya was one of the lucky ones in whose honor our dear friend had donated for the cause. One would rightfully guess I was tearful again. I imagined the scene from the pictures Varun sent, a large playground lit with luminaries at dusk with a big display of light saying 'celebrations.' Quiet prayers, talks and solemn walks around the luminaries created an atmosphere of serenity and reverence, probably lacking in many places of worship with its crowded hustle and bustle.

Feeling grateful I proceeded to shower while Lavanya slumbered with side effects. We always felt that one could never plan enough, so why bother planning actually. On one such useless planning spree, I had optimistically packed enough to last us for three days of hospital stay. I had hoped that the drug would clear within 72 hours, but with that not happening I had told Varun to get me clothes for the next day. If I recall right, my instructions were, "Please get me a denim skirt and a lace top." He brought them and when I went to shower what did I discover! My man had brought my denim skirt and a lace dress!!! The latter a lovely party dress, but definitely not suitable to wear in the hospital! So what does one do! Give very clear instructions the next time. For that particular time, tuck the lace dress into the denim skirt ensuring it didn't stick out from under and go down to get breakfast and coffee hoping that no one saw me as I tried to merge with the walls and walk invisibly into the bistro. We call Murphy's law, Uncle Murphy and as always he was hard at work because I realized that to reach the bistro one had to walk through the building personnel meeting that happened every morning near the winding staircase next to the beautiful grand piano. I still wonder if I was successful in blending in with the walls or were the jokes still on regarding a woman hugging the walls in a weird contraption! The nurses didn't miss an opportunity to rub it into Varun when he came by later in the morning as they chorused, "Just tell when you want your wife to wear her jeans with that dress and skirt!"

They took turns to come in and admire my 'outfit' and consoled me that I looked quite smart indeed! One of them shared her opinion with us saying, "You guys are very good and very positive with the treatment. One mum would get so upset because her child wouldn't clear the drug within 48 or 72 hours that she would move the child to tears." I was aghast. If a child had the capacity, she wouldn't be a patient of leukemia in the first place. I wish parents and care givers would understand that nothing that was happening was the making of the child, parents or anyone else, instead catch that naughty gene which had mutated!

Another mum who couldn't speak English stood outside our door and said to me, "Baby, baby." So I had to say to her, "No no, not a baby but a 15-year-old girl." I had naturally assumed that she asked about Lavanya in the room. The mum again said baby baby, so I thought she asked me if I had more and I tried to explain that I had another, a boy aged 11 years. The woman continued baby baby and pointed to my stomach and I exclaimed no!! No baby. I went in and asked Lavanya's opinion if all the sitting in the hospital had started to make me look round enough to appear pregnant. Lavanya couldn't stop laughing and said that probably the other mum was pregnant. Goodness!! I told Varun that I better hit the treadmill running and Ditto couldn't understand how mum will hit the treadmill running and imagined all possible ways that could be done.

Shilpi shared her moment, "As for babies, I think the most cringing experience I had was when I was being sold a Chinese piece with 100 children embroidered on it to hang in my bedroom for good luck with my forthcoming 'delivery!' Ye lord!"

With that I realized I wasn't alone in those predicaments of sorts. Namrata felt that the blog was the secret formula LOLs, bringing lots of laughter. She visited with reiki, books and things to take the nausea away that had hit with a vengeance. It seemed that our poor girl was bent over the pink basin all the time either throwing up violently or waiting to throw up, though she perked up after Namrata's visit. We tried home remedy of the amazing turmeric plus salt gargles for mouth sores and to protect the food tract from developing sores. The anti-nausea patch behind her ear made her partially blind so she saw us but didn't see us. She tried reading but vision was way too blurred to read, TV watching, too, was out so she lay down through the day, as without eyes there wasn't much she could do. I thought of the visually impaired in the world and felt sad, it was a beautiful world that they couldn't see. We having everything, all working body parts and organs took much for granted. Every day was a lesson.

All roads led to Cupertino. Whoever came to the United States, be it New York, Chicago or San Francisco, they made it a point to detour via Cupertino. We had Surbhi family visiting from Melbourne and Swarnali family from Mumbai. My neighbors Anita and Gina on hearing that we will have company gladly offered their bedrooms in case we ran short of space. I recalled my friend's words about me meeting people only when I put the trash out or how the Aussies were not friendly and the Americans were indifferent. I still marvel at the warmth of the Aussies and the friendliness of the Americans. Nothing that I had been told to expect had happened as both nationalities went out of their way to make newcomers welcome.

What does one do when bored? Our girl lay down with her head on my 'little' stomach and sang songs, nursery rhymes, English as well as French songs – some off key, some melodiously while I lay reading. Every few minutes she would break off and erupt into uncontrollable giggles. Next she would get up and bend over the pink bin to throw up whatever was left in her and resume listening to the music of my stomach. She wondered as to why the stethoscope was invented. There was certainly no need for it because all the doctor needed to do was to put the ears against the patient's tummy to know what was going on. As if in response my tummy made its presence felt by making lot of noises and she had fits of laughter imagining her team of doctors listening to the tummy. Some would need to bend over, others would need to reach, some would stoop and so on, what with some being short and others tall, some fat and others thin, some agile and some clumsy. Visualizing was not only healing but also providing humor.

On days she got bored just being in her hospital room she would phone Joel in Mumbai and make him talk to her for what seemed like forever. The poor guy always obliged and then it was Jayshree's turn in Singapore to hear the laugh and giggles, as without sense of sight the 'laugh senses' seemed to have been heightened. When Varun returned from work he complied to her, "Tell me a story." His stories tend to be pretty repetitive, but she still would listen since childhood with rapt attention. So he began again, "Once upon a time in a place called Redwood City there was a company called Oracle! In Oracle," ... and it went on.

I later apologized to Joel for taking up much of his time in the morning, but he was very kind saying that it was fun talking to her. He described it as a good start to the day. Discussing books, movies and music among other things, especially the part where they tried to figure how many people in the office knew any *One Direction* songs. My sister kept Lavanya company when her health permitted and my brother-in-law spent a lot of time on the phone with her talking random, sensible, nonsense to help her pass that time when nausea let her up. My brother in law's query of, "Do you listen to something, um something, oh yes,

179

something Swift," had her thinking if men really lived in Mars. Clearly his teenagers had introduced him to Taylor Swift, though not very successfully.

Ditto left for New Jersey for Nafis and Lubna's place, with enough excitement to touch the whole neighborhood. Karen, my dear neighbor was around as he was loading his suitcase onto the car and added to his spending money kitty and his joy reached higher limits. United Airlines allowed the dad to see him off till the boarding gate and Nafis was allowed at Newark to wait for him at the gate again. As per rules Varun was required to wait till the flight left the gate and the ground staff shared Ditto's excitement with him as he left. He seemed to have this inane ability to touch everyone around, friends as well as strangers with his innocent enthusiasm. Suddenly there was a vacuum at home; way too silent and Lavanya had only adult company.

Lavanya started taking ginger steps around the house, helped dad cook risotto, graduating to a short walk around the neighborhood. I was actually quite in awe of her confidence and attitude and thanked God for giving her those in plenty. We went for a short walk and met people around and she was comfortable, smiled and spoke to those we met without feeling self-conscious. It was summer so she hadn't started using the lovely caps, scarves that she had received from friends. I thought I was so shallow that I hurried to color my hair when I spotted some grey and there she was almost without hair, acquiring dark spots all over her face, neck and hands, hadn't gone out anywhere except to be admitted or poked and prodded at the hospital for the last four months but hey, had I heard her complain! Hadn't even heard a why me, nor had she asked when that entire saga was going to end.

Lisa's words touched me, "Your children are not just old beautiful souls: they are AMAZING old beautiful souls. And, in the US Midwestern vernacular, them apples don't fall far from the trees. Wow, Lavanya. I have so much to learn from you. I need to come over before the onslaught of guests to massage your shoulders." I shared facts from the treatment as and when they happened and it was beautiful beyond compare to read everyone's thoughts. They came with open minds and love in their hearts that blew not only me away but also others who read their words.

Chapter 25

"Atithi Devo Bhava-
Guests are Gods visiting in another form."
Indian proverb

I had the pleasure of receiving reiki from Namrata to feel rejuvenated and energized. No words could do justice to the heartfelt reiki she did and I would highly recommend periodic reiki session with a good reiki master. I am sure that there are plenty practicing in the big wide world, but there can be few who practiced with the selfless devotion of my friend. I hesitantly did mention compensation as some others had time and again stressed that monetary compensation needed to be involved in healing. In their opinion, the art and science so practiced would be in vain without a fair exchange of forces or energies. She looked at me and smiled to say, "I got to practice on someone who needed it the most – your girl and to see the changes it did to her was more than monetary payment or any other compensation."

She suggested something brilliant while giving reiki to Lavanya. She said that the medicines going into her must be treated as friends, they should be welcomed so they would do what they were supposed to do, kill the leukemia cells and then leave as fast as possible without creating havoc anywhere else. So our new friend was the high dose IV methotrexate, that would remain Lavanya's friend for 24 hours and then would quietly leave. In India the saying of 'Atithi Devo Bhava' translated meant, 'Guests are another form of God visiting,' so I guess if we treated the medicine that way, love it like we love our guests, it could only do right. Lisa loved Namrata's advice and agreed that treating the drug as a friend, the warrior that will do its battle and leave was the way to deal with the situation. She had not known the tradition of viewing visitors as a representation of God and loved the concept. Shilpi, too, loved Namrata's idea and began visualizing our friend coming, having a good time knocking off the required cells candy crush style and then leaving in 24 hours to a huge chorus of cheerful byes! I realized that she was a big fan of candy crush then.

The dose of 'best friend forever' (BFF) methotrexate had been increased to 75% from the previous of 50% of full dose, all the while gauging Lavanya's reactions. When we were not friends with methotrexate earlier, it had caused seizure and knocked her out for a week. I was ready to roll out the red carpet, spread flowers to welcome the drug to do its magic and disappear without a trace. The nurses had begun hydration for our girl at 350 ml per hour to excrete methotrexate at the earliest and that made her hobble to the rest room frequently.

I actually enjoyed my stays with our girl in PEC (Packard at El Camino). As long as she was not sick it served as a time for discovery – me discovering her. I always enjoyed her subtle sense of humor, but with the time I spent with her during treatment I appreciated her great timing and inane ability to laugh at herself first before she commented on anyone. She was most critical of herself aiming for perfection and could joke about that quality, too. She watched as I ate salad with great interest and amusement and observed that I was eating cow food. According to her evolution was going backwards. First man ate raw, then he found fire, followed by cooking and now he was going back to eating raw as more and more people are opting to be vegetarians or including more portions of raw food in their diet. Cows were so much smarter than men. They evolved over time and stuck to eating grass; they even had excellent time management skills. They first ate, to chew and digest later. God gave them four compartments in their stomachs to manage all the skills. Well I never! So I guessed now we knew why we didn't see cows at gyms or even getting a heart surgery. Actually I thought I would ask a vet about that. We let our imagination run wild thinking of humans with compartmentalized tummies but Aparna stopped our imagination all the way from Mumbai reminding us of stomach crunches since we could barely handle one tiny stomach. The humble cow with four compartments in its stomach gained new respect.

With nothing much to do but wait for the friend metho to leave, Lavanya wanted to name the monitors and IV pole and the bags. For some strange reason she wanted to call the IV pole a pig, the big monitor was a donkey, the small monitor was chicken and the bags hanging were cows!! I had no clue as to why, so I asked the reason and it was as follows, though I failed to find the exact connection.

Her cousins in India have this third brother (dare not call him a dog), a Labrador called Scooby. Whenever the stray dogs around the neighborhood needed to be driven away, they would call him and say, "Look Scooby – donkeys." Scooby dear would then bark his head off to drive away the 'donkeys aka stray dogs. So if stray dogs could be donkeys why couldn't some monitor hanging onto a pole be the same! On second thoughts the monitors were quite loud whenever there was bubble in the line and each one had its own distinctive alarm, comparable to irritating barks. The donkey (big monitor) was misbehaving by beeping way too often with some bubble in the line or air in infusion, so we got a whole new donkey.

Mali found the above too cute, a complete new ecosystem in the room. In Alka's words, "Sohini your posts are like sunshine on a cloudy day. Absolutely love your ability to turn negatives into positives, tears to laughter. God bless you all! Always in our thoughts & prayers. Love & blessings!" And I thought hey, I was the mother of the original Miss and Master Sunshine! In Lavanya's friend Yana's words, "Ha-ha-ha, I loved the cow-evolution theory. In fact, there is so much in the world to think about, there are so many things to be explained, but we are always too busy to even stop for a second and ask ourselves any of those interesting questions. Sohini, I think there is another negative that could be turned into positive – you discover your daughter and she discovers the world, from a place that would take the rest of us years to see!"

With the increase in dose, Lavanya started waking up due to nausea. I couldn't begin to imagine seeing a loved one wake up from slumber because of sickness or nausea and here I was seeing her wracked with nausea, vomiting with huge shudders shaking not only her but also me to the core. The nurse gave her a sedative and I waited for it to kick in. Lavanya's Chemistry teacher Mia Onodera had said to her at the time of diagnosis, "You will really get to know your parents now and them you." I so agreed, facets unknown to me about her came to light, with great personality traits hidden in daily living, emerging in the bedridden constrained times. We had many conversations, some of which made me think deep, others made me laugh and many where I drew blanks. The teen mind jostled with mine to look at life from different angles and I appreciated the new angles.

At that point I had nothing new to report except that the animals in the room were steadily increasing. So we had adjectives prefixed to them like, good donkey, bad donkey, nice cow, mad cow, etc. The bed was the worst donkey ever as it wasn't as firm as she would have liked. The hospital massage therapist worked on her aching joints and muscles. Then the chaplain in the hospital heard about this teen in great pain and nausea and came by to pray for her aches to disappear. We had met the chaplain in the Stanford branch of the hospital and he was aware that we respected all faiths but the one in El Camino branch had not met us and hence wasn't aware of our thoughts. I loved what she did. It never fails to amaze me that everyone does his or her homework before visiting a patient/caregiver/family. She explained that while she prayed for us in the chapel she would like to pray the Hindu way, too. So she went through some books and brought us some writings from Hindu scriptures and traditions. I told her that she could continue to pray however and wherever she wanted for our girl. It was the prayer that mattered not the who, how, where, when or to whom. Nevertheless, the little thoughts went a long way in strengthening one's belief in the goodness of mankind. I do wonder now as to why the word 'womankind' is not used!

Some said they read our blog first thing on waking up squinting their eyes without glasses and many said they read it last before they slept. I thought that there might be times when the reader would go back and forth in our lives because some of the thoughts were related to what happened before but at the end it's the story of a young girl, a teen whose life changed with the disease, towards better, making her a stronger individual with inherent compassion and maturity lacking in many adults. As life folded from that day of diagnosis on March 26th 2013, we learned as individuals, grew as a family and appreciated so much more than what would have been possible had normal life just passed us. It made us better individuals. Some are blessed because they are beautiful individuals without life's experiences and some learn to improve with life's experience. Even today I learn something new from everyone around me and feel very privileged to have those impressionable individuals in our lives, who impacted us positively, and continue to do so constantly. I couldn't begin to describe what our friends did for us. At the cost of sounding cliché their actions and words had become therapeutic, plus the blog had become an excellent source of review of past episodes of low counts, aches, the goods and the bads. Since it was pretty much chronologically written anything we wished to check about what reaction happened when, its extent and how, was all in there like an open diary.

We kept the visualization on for methotrexate leaving happily and hurriedly. I pondered over, "Your beliefs become your thoughts, your thoughts become your words, your words become your actions, your action becomes your habits, your habits become your values and your values become your destiny." Now before anyone could commend my writing I had to let everyone know that those are words of Mahatma Gandhi and not mine.

Chapter 26

"You can't have a good day with a bad attitude and you can't have a bad day with a good attitude."

Unknown

We couldn't stop smiling as our dear friends from Melbourne arrived. We had an oh so Bollywood reunion. Had that been filmed Bollywood style there would have been music, violin, flowers floating down as friends ran across the car park in slow motion lugging suitcase and flowers to hug, laugh, cry all at the same time. Lavanya walked with her animal farm in tow to the entrance of the hospital while Swarnali and Srey ran as fast as they could. The afternoon flew by amidst chats, games and giggles. Lavanya looked so crestfallen as they left in the evening that they decided to visit her again the following day before leaving for airport and thereafter Surbhi family was landing from Melbourne.

The icing on cake was when my brother-in-law called to share that my older nephew had at that moment completed a 12-hour long interview starting with a written test, group discussion, technical rounds, ending with HR (Human Resources) rounds to get his dream job. Thereby I became the aunt of an engineer who was going to work exactly where he had wanted, going to prove yet again that when you want something really bad the world conspires to get it for you. I did thank God that when we were looking for work after grad school all those years ago interviews were much simpler and shorter. All my school friends readily, whole-heartedly agreed. God had been very kind to us by making us a 1960s child ...

Madam M, not to be confused with Judi Dench in James Bond, was the new name for methotrexate and she finally left! We attributed the wonderful luck to Jhoomar who had walked in with her thermos full of rejuvenating tea. However, just as Lavanya got ready to wear her shoes she found she couldn't put her feet in. Her big toe was all swollen and there was a faint yellow mark around the nail that turned out to be pus, an infection. Something painful but negligible for you and me, but for her it could mean 2 weeks in the hospital with IV antibiotics. Since the discharge was already signed onto the computer we were packed off to the ER.

The numbing cream lidocaine was applied and we waited for it to take affect for blood draw to check her counts again as the pus needed to be drained. It was not creditable but I realized then that I would come to know when a blood draw would be eventful and when peaceful and it was not a nice feeling when you knew that it was going to be the former. The saving grace was that Varun was there to hold her as the nurse tried accessing and failed. I thought that she missed the port because when she probed, Lavanya screamed and the mean mum put a stop to it resulting in a dirty look and the end of attempt.

The nurse must have gone and cried blue murder against me because the head nurse came bustling in and said in a loud authoritative voice to our girl, "Now, if you were my child I would not put you through accessing, but insist on a peripheral blood draw to avoid causing infection by accessing the port time and again just for a CBC (Complete Blood Count)."

Probably to make a point she said that some four times, slightly louder every time. I too drew myself to my full 5 ft. 4 inches of height and told her that well, she was 'my' child and I would not like her to be probed time and again as her veins couldn't be found. She insisted that they were experts and we said Stanford, too, had experts who probed for 6 hours without luck, not to blame anyone but only the thin stubborn veins. At Stanford they had very thoughtfully drawn veins with a marker on her arms and legs with the aid of an ultra sound machine to help in finding veins the first time we were admitted way back in March. She requested for one poke. We agreed for one poke but no probe. I think the poke was okay but it was the probe within the vein that hurt. When the needle went in smoothly and the blood was drawn it was easy but when the needle went in and no blood could be drawn, the interior probe with the needle to find the elusive vein would begin. I felt sickened to see the needle inside the vein being maneuvered to get blood and I refused to have that done on our child who was already living the nightmare associated with cancer treatment. A nurse came and tied the band, felt and felt some more with no luck. Thankfully they stuck to their promise of one poke and she didn't even try poking till she got a vein and called another nurse to try. This other nurse came, again all masked and covered to start with the same process of tying the band, beating the hand, putting warm packs to make the veins prominent, etc. By then Lavanya was traumatized and was shaking, shivering, crying while Varun held her. I told her in our language, Hindi, that the new lady seemed confident and would successfully draw blood with one poke. To my surprise and embarrassment, the lady replied back in the same language, that yes, she would and promised to be gentle or nothing. She was extraordinarily gentle and she did it! Blood from vein and not from port at the first attempt! The counts were good; pus was drained and sent for culture. No IV antibiotics were needed, but ten days of oral antibiotics were prescribed and by the time we reached home it was very late. In Macarena's words, "Dear Lavanya this brings back all my memories of blood draws and port access and having a new port inserted as my weird vascular system decided to disconnect itself!! I found deep visualization helped. Just before I was touched I would tell the nurse I was going to my beach and just as I was being poked we talked about our favorite beaches and vacations!! Hope this helps." Macarena had been there and done that with her breast cancer treatment so could empathize with Lavanya much more than anyone else.

I must admit that during instances like these I sometimes reverted to speaking in Hindi to the family against our own unspoken rules of no private talks in Hindi in public out of politeness and respect. At instances like these, I again admit that I didn't say very complimentary things in Hindi. It went more like let the wicked witch do her work and disappear and things on those lines with all due apologies to all concerned. It was said in zest, just to bring a smile onto our girl's face as she heard mum talking nonsense. It wasn't meant to be mean to anyone. Well in this instance I was so glad I didn't revert to that kind of humor as the lady turned out to be Indian, her gown, mask, goggles and cap covered most of her so we knew only when she spoke the language that she had similar origin as us! Surely she wouldn't have appreciated the mother of the patient calling her wicked witch, zest or not!

Ditto returned from Lubna and Nafis's home armed with presents from them as well as what he bought with his 'own' money. When he arrived home with Varun, he was endearingly like his dad in everything he did. First things first, he unpacked and showered, after giving us all our presents of course. What touched me most that he had brought a present for my neighbor Karen who had given him spending money when he was leaving. If it were possible, I loved him more for that.

Meanwhile the pus increased so surgical intervention was necessary. As I said earlier, what may be a minor incident for you and me, can become a major issue for a leukemia patient if not monitored closely. While the doctors contemplated on IV or oral antibiotic intervention Lavanya made me plead with them for oral drugs rather than IV as she didn't feel too sick and it was ahem, her mother's birthday. I almost went underground with embarrassment, as a grown up forty plus woman telling the doctors, "Eh, ahem you see, um it is my birthday and I want to celebrate it with my daughter and the rest of the family at home." Ah the joys of motherhood!

I thought that exactly a year ago, on this very day, we were three days old in the States, complete strangers in a new city, staying in a hotel, preparing to move into the house, missing Melbourne, Mumbai, family, friends and all things familiar. What a contrast it was today! With a shared journey of Lavanya's recovery, we had moved closer to those far away, made new friends closer to home and discovered a world more beautiful than we had ever known. The disease has brought us closer together within family/friends, made us recognize deeply rooted thoughts and values and the blog that started as an update on our girl's treatment had become our biggest source of support. Driving with these thoughts playing on my mind I reached home to find two parcels. One was a huge bouquet all the way from Singapore!! Had I even tried I couldn't have thanked Shilpi enough for giving me a beautiful end to the day. They were absolutely gorgeous and I was very touched. The bouquet even carried a little note, "I have travelled from far, put me in water with the first packet and I will bloom in 12 hours, add second packet after three days and watch me stay." In the days of smart phones, we had smart flowers too!

Hubby dear had pre-ordered a cake which was picked up on the way back from work. He had thought all my angels would be there so it was big enough to feed an army. And yeah, all the angels did turn up, no invitation issued, none expected and we all glowed in the warmth of family and friends, feeling loved, cherished and blessed.

Chapter 27

"If you don't understand how a woman could both love her sister dearly and want to wring her neck at the same time, then you were probably an only child."

Linda Sunshine

The child life department at the hospital told us that they were organizing a day trip for its teen onco patients – a day filled with pampering at a spa followed by lunch at Santana Row. They were to be chauffeured in a pink limo from the hospital to the spa, followed by lunch and back. Lavanya was in two minds about the trip imagining herself in the bright 'pink limo,' not exactly her idea of fun and also the fact that she wouldn't know anyone, but then the spa beckoned. I thought only a mum would say what I did to help her make up her mind, "It's only a day trip with 11 other girls, not exactly spending a lifetime with them." So yes, at 8.00 a.m. we were to drop our girl to the hospital and she would be back at 4.00 p.m. to be picked up again from there. A hospital visit sans a visit within, a visit without pokes, prods, blood draws, labs, access and de-access. She would get to choose three out of the four options offered – manicure, pedicure, massage and facial, while make-up was done for all. Hairstyling wasn't included as most of the girls were in various stages of hair loss/gain.

It was indeed strange that for a while, at any given time the family couldn't rejoice entirely. I believed that by the grace of God, our families' and friends' combined prayers, our girl was responding well, having fewer side effects and was going forward to a bigger cocktail of drugs in the coming weeks. However, my sister who had been keeping ill health for almost a year had to be hospitalized yet again. Till then she and Lavanya had been playing seesaw with hospital visits and my sister's end looked low at that moment. We had been talking to her and my brother-in-law every day and were waiting for her complete recovery to rejoice as a family.

My sister was supposed to be having a blood infection and hence her counts were going up and down. Then the diagnosis came that it was Myelodysplastic Syndrome, a disease of the elderly where the bone marrow didn't produce enough healthy cells. No one had an answer as to how my normal healthy happy 51 years old sister got the disease affecting those above 65. We were to be admitted for the next round of Madam M visit with a cocktail of drugs with lumbar puncture followed by transfer by ambulance for the rest of the IV drug. My sister was admitted to ICU due to her slow response to treatment for her bone marrow disorder. Mali went in for surgery to remove her malignant body part and was promised discharge in a couple of days. Heavens be praised! When my mum was operated for the same, she was in the hospital for more than a week, but then that was 1995 in a small city called Nagpur in India. Medical science deserved all praises for coming far.

We checked into Stanford for the lumbar puncture. Father and daughter went for a walk and she paused in front of a door that said 'Board Room' and joked if the name was acquired due to the boredom it generated. Once she was exhausted we continued our wait at the reception and saw a young man walking in and the ladies at the reception 'ooohed' and 'aahed' then continued conversing with him like old buddies. When I was called to be informed of our turn I overheard them asking him, "And where is mum?" And he beamed, "Oh now I drive, I drove myself today." So, this young man was a patient just like our girl a few years ago, driven to and fro by either mum or dad for his checkup and chemotherapy. Now fully cured he drove himself for his yearly checkup. I, at once started daydreaming that few years on Lavanya would drive herself, beaming to say – "Yes, I drove in myself today," and yet another mum present there would get a boost in her confidence, hope and belief.

News came from my brother-in-law that my sister was put on life support due to multiple organ failure. Varun immediately booked me on the shortest possible route to reach her at the earliest, flying out of San Francisco via Beijing and Bangkok to reach Kolkata in less than 24 hours, with return after a week. It did seem kind of crazy but the other usual routes would take 30 plus hours. At that point I didn't know really what to think, pray and wish for. I always inculcated positive thoughts against all odds and I had immense support from my family and friends but this was straight out of a bad novel/movie, something quite unreal. Fervent prayers were on for Madam M to leave at the earliest so that I could leave without worries. I had not one or two but three rocks at home – my hubby and kids and I knew they will pull through the week's hospitalization and treatment.

Suddenly I was blank. What could I say? What was I supposed to think and do? I was torn between my first-born and my only sibling, the only surviving member from the family I was born in! How I wished that the family I was born into and the family I gave birth to could be together. The more I thought, the more blanks I faced. Did I thank God that my sister had a doctor who was by her bedside almost 24/7 trying everything he could to save her, calling in specialists from everywhere to see her, even becoming a donor of blood products while he treated her? Or did I thank God for giving her a husband who was being so brave and strong as he saw her slipping away or her older boy who stood by her helpless, with the younger one reaching from college within the next 12 hours. Then I thought probably I should thank God for Varun, who without another thought looked up airlines and the shortest route to reach India, or the kids who told me to go and be with her. It felt very clichéd to say tough times don't last but tough people do, because none of us are that tough after all.

My sister's condition continued to deteriorate and I wondered if I would make it on time. The plan was to go direct to the hospital from the airport sometime in the middle of the night on arrival. I imagined myself sitting at her hospital bed, just like I sit with Lavanya, chatting and laughing. I thought focusing on visualization had helped us with our girl and it will help with my sister, too. When I spoke to Dr Dahl about my sister and current circumstances, my faith in the goodness of humanity reached newer heights. He said that it sure was a bummer of a time. He could discharge Lavanya with her levels going down as per requirement, but with the onset of fever he couldn't until blood and urine culture results came. He tried to make things easier for the dad and kids, with me gone. He put in a note to hospital management explaining the situation requesting that the family be allowed to stay together in our girl's room. That meant Ditto, too, got a bed with Lavanya in the room and Varun had the parent's bed already. With my departure, Varun would take on 24-hour vigil by her bedside. I sent up a silent prayer yet again. While we did have our dear friends who would have gladly adopted Ditto for those few days, it made us feel better having each other around.

Achala wrote that if it were possible her thoughts were with us even more. She, too, has two sisters and could empathize and feel for me. She sent me a virtual hug as she wrapped her arm around me and blessed the doctor and hospital staff for the accommodation they were providing at the time of need. Jayshree, Shilpi, Alka, Mary Jane, Macarena were joined by others with everyone having similar thoughts in their minds, similar prayers echoing in their hearts. In Lisa's words, "Sohini, I wish you safety, strength and a squadron of angels on your travels, both physically and spiritually, to your sister's side. The miracle is you, Varun, Ditto and Lavanya: a most miraculous God-reflecting family of spirits. May the angels lift and protect all of you in the coming days." Priya Devotta wrote, "Sohini, I know it's easy for me to say, 'stay strong, keep your faith' and so many other inspirational words, but I have not walked a day in your shoes, but believe me when I say, I admire you, your strength and for all the speed bumps in your path, your grit at being able to see so much positivity in everything & continually taking that step forward. We cannot as humans fathom the whys for what comes our way, but continue to support you through my prayers & pray specially to keep you mentally, physically, emotionally & spiritually strong, to be the role model that you have become to all of us. Praying for all of God's angels to surround all of you in the coming days. Praying for all of you."

With tight hugs to Lavanya, Varun, Ditto, everyone's wishes in my mind and all the prayers in my heart I boarded the long flight to Kolkata.

Chapter 28

*"If you have a sister and she dies, do you stop saying
you have one? Or are you always a sister, even when the
other half of the equation is gone?"*

Jodi Picoult

We were in disbelief ... in denial ... in shock! I didn't make
it on time. The doctors did their best to keep her, at least for
me to say goodbye to her, but maybe she wished for relief
from pain and passed away of a cardiac arrest 12 hours
before I landed. As per Hindu rites she was cremated and I
stay grateful to my brother-in-law and their boys as they
waited for my arrival. I got to see her mortal remains to
wish her a peaceful, joyful journey above and beyond.
Friends, neighbors, her farm hands, everyone, including her
dog walker came to bid the loving soul adieu.

I couldn't imagine that my last link to our beautiful
childhood was gone, my last connection to our maiden

name Banerjee had left way before her time and I had no one to share those special, silly, funny moments, memories to reminisce about any more. Third time in a row I was making that very long flight, first for mum, then dad and now for dear sis, ironically all in August. I thought that they might be having a party up there while I carried on in shock and disbelief. The death of someone who has lived his or her life to a ripe old age causes grief but when the loss is of someone in the prime of his or her life, that grief is combined with disbelief, an ache in heart that the ever-trusted time too is unable to heal. I recall that funerals in Ghana were a huge celebration with the burial casket being planned in the lifetime of a person with lot of enthusiasm and thought. They bid their elders a warm fond farewell but I couldn't bring myself to bid my sibling the same. A life gone in a breath! I wished for the three of my family members to rock on in heaven and to my dear sister I said to go joyfully, go peacefully, go knowing that you were much loved, are and would always be loved and missed every day.

Our circle was in a similar state of shock, disbelief and sorrow and we received overwhelming love and affection mourning the death of a beautiful person. No one could imagine what we were going through and I didn't wish anyone to know either. 51 years of age was no age to leave this beautiful world. It was an age, in fact to continue working hard, look back at life with peace and happiness, enjoy the visits of your children who are settled and doing well in life, reap the rewards of your hard work, sit in that chair sipping a cup of tea with your partner waiting for the day to begin, watch the sunset with a wine, sleep with a contentment that yes, you had achieved much as a person, had done good and you were at peace with yourself and with the world. I wished she could have seen her boys going to work, getting married, had enjoyed being a grandma. We believe that the soul lives on so I assume she would experience all of the above, only without our awareness.

Her dog Scooby refused to budge from the front door of their home needing to be fed and taken care of like an infant. His continued vigil reminded us of Hachiko, the dog in Tokyo that waited for his master at Shibuya railway station. After all the ceremonies, a beautiful picture of her smiling her radiant smile was garlanded with fragrant roses and kept on the mantle. Scooby thereafter parked himself in front of the picture, paws in front, continuing the wait.

During my short stay in Kolkata, I received an amazing surprise, one of a kind when my two dear friends arrived for just a day from Singapore to hold my hand. Shilpi, my friend from high school and Jayshree, my one-time neighbor connected from the blog in Singapore and flew in together, moving all beyond words while the rest of our buddies continued keeping us in their cloak of love.

Back home in Cupertino, Lavanya and Varun met Mr. Hicks to work out her schedule to accommodate chemo with classes. There was only one word for him and the school- incredible! They were marvelous with their level of understanding and co-operation going above and beyond our imagination and expectation. They thought of aspects we hadn't thought, had information we hadn't known was available. I had bought a book by Louis Hay called *You Can Heal Yourself* for my Brother in law. I read it before I gave it to him. The book asked, how do you see people around you? I thought, 'Just beautiful,' and that was the beginning of the healing process – with beauty around. Lisa thought that this ability to recognize beauty and feel gratitude would bring out the best within and those around us. I agreed that gratitude and love went around, the more you give the more you get. If you give without expectations, you will be surprised by the bountiful you receive.

My brother-in-law had gone back to work, as he couldn't imagine staying home in her absence, feeling worse. Though come dinnertime the three of us would sit at the table, my bro-in-law, my nephew and I, feeling lost in her absence. One empty chair made all the difference. I told them stories of our childhood that were fun ways to remember her, rather than in her sickness. He, too, had kept all the pictures of her healthy days around so he remembered her in good health and happier times.

She was seven years my senior, but was naïve like a 17-year-old, the true Bengali of the two of us, with culinary skills to salivate a seasoned master chef. She was a mum, a daughter, a daughter-in-law, a wife and a sister before she was an individual. I told them how she was the religious one. I, probably aged fourteen then, and the prankster in the family had marked her face with red lipstick while she slept. On waking up she was thrilled, thinking she had been blessed by God almighty as we Indians apply red vermillion when visiting temple. The simpleton thought that temple visited her while she slept. She also was the perpetually foot in the mouth one. On her high school graduation, everyone including parents, uncles, aunts, grandparents wanted to know her plans there on. To everyone's consternation she had gleefully replied, "Aami BIYE korbo." While everyone thought that she meant to marry as that is what 'biye' meant in our language, but she of course meant B.A., the Bachelor of Arts kind of B.A.! She was my confidante, caretaker and protector. Anything wrong that I would do, forget things at school, get someone else's bag home instead of mine, yep, I could do that too, forget to take things to school from home, oh she rescued me from all of those. She also was the sensitive one as every year visiting our grandparents in Banaras and Delhi during summer vacation, to the embarrassment of our parents their younger daughter would practically dance her way back, happy to be going home, but the older one compensated that lack of sensitivity by sobbing her heart out all the way to the airport or railway station. Now that I have kids of my own I realized why God made siblings so different despite similar genes. Siblings balance the family with their usually contrasting personalities, bringing out the best in each other. Aparna understood about the differences in the nature of siblings as she had a brother who was completely different from her and her two daughters differed from each other like chalk and cheese. She completely understood what I meant. Rachna Palit warmed us by pointing out that we were blessed since we realized that we had beauty around us. People worked hard to reach that space where only beauty surrounded them but we were lucky, as we had attained that elusive space. People dealt with losses in their own personal ways and our way was beautiful, because we reminisced about good times, looking back with fondness and love, but not with grief, regret or anger.

Lavanya had promised herself that she would attend school from day one, but couldn't due to a whole day chemo appointment. It broke my heart to see her quiet, resigned acceptance of the situation. That promise of attending the first day of school after summer couldn't be kept under the circumstances, and she quietly consoled herself, "If not the first day, then I will attend school from day two." On return from India, I found her very upbeat as she had attended a day of school by then and with a spring in her step she kept repeating – "I went to school, I went to school, I am going to school again tomorrow." The efficiency with which my family had tended to themselves in my absence had me proud.

Both our children appeared ill at ease as to what to say to me to console. Both had been always pampered and much loved by their beloved masi/mashi/aunt. In Indian language, Hindi, 'ma' is mother while 'si' meant 'like' making 'masi' 'like mum' so basically aunt signified someone like mum. Though I would say the masi/aunt had the pleasure of only loving and pampering while disciplining was the mum's forte. They hugged me, peered at me and then continued to share all that happened in past one week that I was away. I kept getting glances from them from time to time and Ditto the sensitive one, especially kept an eye out for any sniffs. I couldn't even sniff the normal sniff without him rushing to me to ask if I was okay. He just warmed my heart every minute, every day.

I felt sorry for those I met when I went around my day-to-day affair. Whatever happens, ironically and beautifully, life does go on. Many of those I met looked a little surprised to see me going about normal routine, a few remarked that I looked great considering I was sad, jetlagged and grieving the loss of a sister. I so understood what they meant and empathized with their thoughts of confusion as to how to behave around me. I think grief is a personal feeling. Some go into hiding, some bawl, some shed silent tears, a few talk and others go mum while many others put on an act that everything was normal. Some even vent anger and stronger emotions. I don't know which category we fell into, probably a bit of all of them. Someone asked me as to how I was handling the situation. I was at a loss and thought well, since one could not plan to handle such a situation, God forbid when it happened, one did what one had to or could do. Christine agreed that I had rightly captured the difficulties that come with loss from both the perspective of the onlooker and the mourner. It was such an uncertain and ever-changing situation as we journey through those days, months after losing a cherished soul.

Chapter 29

The rounds of chemo were leaving Lavanya exhausted with constant fatigue and nausea. While waiting for the next episode of friend metho to leave, Lavanya thought that she had had enough of the treatment and wished to opt out of the regime as she felt better with the disease without the diagnosis than with the diagnosis and treatment. All I could say that while my feelings were the same, the treatment was known to be traumatic and she had coped with much courage and resilience. A few years from now I hoped to look back at this period as a bad dream that left us stronger and closer.

I thought of pulling through this time of grief by finding joy in everything I could. One of the greatest joy was achieved from a beautiful thought. Ditto surprised me by saying, "Mummy, can you take me shopping?" Now that was a statement that came usually from Lavanya, so, amused, I asked him what he wished to shop. His reply warmed me from my heart right down to my toes. "I know you feel sad as Mashi is no more and I want to make you happy by cooking you a meal, a meal of jasmine rice and teriyaki chicken. You need to take me to the supermarket to buy the ingredients; I gave him a big fat hug, and promised to take him shopping.

Surprise of surprises that even the terribly tough technology brought me joy. I was talking to Varun about all the mails I had received while in India. Amongst them were a few from my next-door neighbor Gina. She wrote that she saw our home in darkness and hence knew that Varun was not back with the kids from the hospital and she prayed for a quick discharge. My hubby thought about the darkness in the house and didn't like the idea of me returning to it and did some technological improvisation. No, he didn't get sensor lights or the timed lights. To switch on these lights, I didn't have to physically switch them on nor did anyone have to walk by for the sensors to be activated for the lights to come on. These were smart lights and had their own iPhone app. They came on either by me sending a mail to Varun titled lights on or they could come on anytime I used the iPhone app to switch on the colors I wanted. Warm white, yellow, disco, beach, relaxing, reading and so on. Cutting a long story short the lights now could be switched on from anywhere in the world, the next room or from ten minutes' drive away. Many might be aware of this app but to me, a tech novice, this was sheer genius as well as funny.

I sent him many mails to see how the system worked and was chuffed to note it worked every time with superb precision. We found joy in the simplicity of routine when Lavanya went to school for three consecutive days, climbed stairs albeit slowly, did homework on return home and ate normally without feeling nauseous.

While admitted in the hospital for methotrexate to clear Lavanya's system, we pretty much followed the same routine every day and night. With all medicines done by 9.30 p.m. I would sit by her bed with the lights dimmed and she would look at me with her big beautiful eyes asking for stories. I told her plenty, quite different from those I told her as a baby. Now the stories were of my childhood, her childhood and we fondly remembered Ditto's. I recalled my days of visiting grandparents, both maternal and paternal every summer. The early morning dip with my sister and cousins in the holy Ganges flowing close to the house and eating sweets and samosa on our way back, my grandfather's pet tortoise, grandma's pet parrot who yapped the whole day long asking for tea and her dog who loved to snuggle. We laughed over Ditto's baby time queries whether he sat with an umbrella while he was in my tummy to protect himself from all the food that I ate which might have fallen on him or why 'yoghurt' was not 'myghurt', likewise for 'Europe and Myrope'. We both laughed aloud remembering his question of "Where is cardadad, why do you use only cardamom in desserts?" and giggled uncontrollably on his suggestion of changing his name to October, his birth month, since he had friends named April, May and June in school. He was profound at times, wondering if God recycled souls or was there an equivalent of washing machine in heaven to cleanse them before sending them back to earth. He gave thinking outside the box a whole new dimension.

It was close to full moon and I would see the movement of the moon across the window of the hospital room from the same spot every night. I would tell her that by the time the moon reached the end of the window we would be discharged and be home where we would see the moon from our bedroom windows, which would be definitely more pleasurable.

It gave me goose bumps to think that was the fastest discharge Lavanya had had and that, too, with a full 100 percent dose. Our representatives in heaven were surely working hard. I also pinched myself to make me believe that we were almost towards the end of the third major phase of the treatment. Methotrexate was known to cause treatment delays with neurological issues requiring long gaps between doses and I thanked God for blessing us with clockwork precision methotrexate. Varun teased me that it followed punctuality just like yours truly. I confess I do have a bad rep in our friends' circle. While everyone would be given the time of 7.00 p.m. to turn up for dinner, I would be told 8.00 p.m., eventually everyone turning up at 8.00 p.m. with precision. I clearly didn't follow the Indian Standard Time that was infamous in its unpunctuality.

When Lavanya was a baby Varun was posted in Kingston, Jamaica and she started speaking a few words there. I wondered if anyone outside of Jamaica was aware that most Jamaicans didn't say the letter 'h.' The letter 'o' replaced the letter 'h' in their vocabulary. So in their case Om was where the art was (home is where the heart is) and that there is always hope, you bet there is hope always. Home has the word OM in it so no wonder it is a special place and as a baby she did call it OM. Lavanya would keep murmuring during her painful trance, "Mommy, I want to go home," and Namrata would say, "You will go home surely, just because you keep chanting 'OM'." We did head Om thereafter. Lisa felt that everyone could convert to the 'OM' experience to reach a level of goodness that could be associated with it.

Soon after Lavanya's discharge Prema and Snegha arrived from Chicago. I teared up as I watched Prema with our children, doing the things my sister would have done. Making their favorite meals, giving that much loved head massage. My sister loved pampering and loving our kids and I felt her absence much more than ever. My brother-in-law put up her picture on the wall (the real wall of their home, not FB wall) alongside our dear departed mum and dad and he, too, wondered about this life we have, family we cherish, only to go away leaving behind people with their memories. Radhika, who studied about past life regression said that we are with the same set of people in every birth and that gave me something to look forward to because we were blessed with a wonderful family and circle of friends. Achala felt honored to be included in our daily life and Jayshree wrote that she looked forward to being there in every life, if the past life regression theory was to be believed. We would know each other in every life in different capacities. I selfishly hoped for the same husband, daughter, son, friends and family. I wonder if they were cringing at the thought!!

213

We took Prema and Snegha to see the Golden Gate Bridge, Pier 39 and drive around San Francisco. To see Lavanya enjoying an ice cream cone sitting by Pier 39 listening to the sea lions roar, watching the tiny specs of sailboats on the waves, her newly grown scanty hair blowing in the wind was a sight we would treasure for a long time. Someone had said to me that we must have been missing normal life of doing the mundane above things and I thought over it. Did we really miss it? Surprisingly the answer was a no, a happy no, perhaps because we were so focused on our goal of getting our girl treated and cured that everything else was secondary and I thanked God every day for giving us the fortitude and ability to do so. We cherished those scattered opportunities but never lamented that they didn't happen often enough. As a family combined with our friends circle we stood united in our goal, the same group of people who were supposed to be coming along with us from many lives and will do for many lives.

The hospital held some activities for the in-patients and Lavanya joined a session of making soaps with glycerin and fragrance. That gave birth to an unending interest in soap making, so much so that after a year of that one session in the hospital she launched her own online soap-selling business, the proceeds from which were divided between leukemia research in Stanford and Leukemia and Lymphoma Society. She graduated to making themed soaps, with someone ordering soaps for a baby shower. Lubna ordered for Eid and Stanford Children's Hospital gave her space to put up stall for Christmas. She made soaps shaped like Christmas tree, ones that looked like candy cane, ginger bread man, snowflake, cookies and twirls. Google gave her unending options and she enthusiastically tried many. I made many trips to Michaels the hobby shop to get glycerin. Ditto helped her to cut and melt glycerin while dad cut her soap loaf into perfect little rectangles. Our wonderful friends from everywhere supported as always by placing orders for birthdays, anniversaries, Christmas and hostess gifts. Achala decided she would present everyone with soaps from then on. We were all with her in her crusade against cancer in every way.

Chapter 30

"Everything you can imagine is real."

Pablo Picasso

The above was said decades ago signifying that there is a possibility of converting our imagination into reality. I believe after much research now in the 21st century it is called visualization. We all thought, imagined and visualized a smooth phase of treatment and I was thrilled that we completed a difficult stage of treatment without hiccups or delays.

Lavanya was feeling good, looking great, appetite was almost back, handwriting was improving, posture and gait were better, energy levels were higher and she was happy where she was. God is truly great. The doctors were happy with her reports and felt that she was headed in the right direction. She was good to start the next phase of treatment called Interim Maintenance 2 followed by Delayed

Intensification (again, I wonder who names them). One of the drugs was known to weaken the heart muscles so an Echo Cardiogram was requested prior to beginning.

Amidst all treatment planning and scheduling Lavanya asked the doctor as to how she would be around mid Oct, as 17th Oct would see her turning 16. Well, unless she got neutropenia and was admitted she would be fine to party away from hospital. I had to smile to myself as she dragged me to her room to show me all the homework and assignments completed. After seeing and hearing all the school excitement I excused myself saying, "I spent the whole day with you, Lavanya, now I will go and spend some time with daddy." Her reply made me think that not too many mums were in that enviable situation as me – "It's only 9 p.m. now, Mum, and the day has not ended. It will end at midnight, only for the next day to begin so ... " So yes, I would gladly spend more time in her room and the only way she would shoo me out was when I started clearing her table and as expected she shooed me out the moment I began that.

Days went by to become weeks, my posts on our blog reduced with Lavanya settling into therapy. Varun and I resumed our evening walks around the block. We were confident enough to leave Lavanya with Ditto for 45 minutes. The best sounds we would hear on return were many and each day different though just as beautiful as the previous. The most amusing was when we overheard the kids playing a game of SIMMS together and discussing whether the newborn baby in the game should be a werewolf or a witch. Gone were the days when in games a newborn could either be a girl or a boy. Then over the

217

weekend on return from yet another walk found both of them hard at work, she dictating and he typing her homework as her fingers had neuropathy. That she is able to do AP (Advanced Placement) homework with other homework of endless hours over the weekend itself spoke a lot about her determination and enthusiasm but the beauty of it was the joy with which it was done and the greater happiness that was derived from the accomplishment of completing it all.

When the chemotherapy made writing difficult she requested her doctors for a slightly reduced dose. The oncologist wished her to receive the best treatment with highest possible dose to reduce the chances of relapse while she wanted to have a life beyond cancer and chemotherapy. Though for her, life didn't require too much, in her words – "I just want to be able to hold my pen and write." The 100% dose of medicines didn't allow her to do that. The oncologist and patient reached a balance where both were happy, she could work and he thought she was receiving a dose that was good for her.

She went back to school. I would love to have been there to see the sights of her teachers from Sophomore year welcoming her back to school with so much love and hugs that my otherwise quiet girl felt and reflected a warmth to last her for days thereafter. The silent starlit night, Ditto practicing clarinet while I wound up the kitchen for the night, Varun giving her ever painful back a massage while she looked blissful though complaining that Ditto's clarinet 'noises' were highly disturbing, are few of the things I will probably recollect fondly when I am all grey and wrinkled.

Not that I am not grey and un-wrinkled now, but let's say when they become more evident.

Malini had her surgery, was healed, even hosted a small party for welcoming Ganesha for the auspicious occasion of, let's call his birthday, (The Indians know about Ganesh Chaturthi and Gauri Pooja, haldi kum kum). In fact, when we visited her we were amazed to see her happily cleaning her house after a round of chemotherapy. We then knew how superman and other heroes/heroines, etc. came into existence ... they had won over cancer.

Even we did our prayers to welcome Ganesha and I made sweets called besan laddoo, which are basically balls of roasted gram flour mixed with powdered sugar and clarified butter/ghee. They look like yellow or brown balls and I watched with much amusement when Lavanya took the yolks of boiled eggs I had set aside for breakfast and arranged them nicely on a plate to call out to her brother, "Ditto come and eat laddoos." Our original sweet tooth came jumping up the steps and looked suspiciously at the greyish yellow 'laddoos.' I thought siblings of all generations are the same. I had given my sister a teaspoon of vanilla essence to drink saying it was holy water called 'charanamrit' when I was probably Lavanya's age. It smells amazing but the taste of vanilla essence is ... Well try it! It is bad and it amazes me that something that tastes so bad has that amazing flavor and aroma.

With these scattered little incidents of fun and laughter I realized that adversities made one stronger, more appreciative of things in and around, bringing a clarity that might be missed under normal circumstances. The difference could be seen in all aspects of life be it in the

219

attitude or caring concerns of nurses who had been patients themselves as opposed to those who had not and that was just one example. I had read about one of the greatest Presidents of America, President Roosevelt became a better, more compassionate person after he was affected by polio. Personally, I became a more patient person and I was a willing listener rather than a talker, though to be fair I should let my family determine this.

Lavanya always preferred the drugs to be injected slowly into her port as the proximity of the port near her throat gave her the taste of saline, heparin and everything that was injected and they didn't taste good. A nurse asked her if she wanted to push the saline, heparin herself because in her experience when the kids pushed it in themselves they didn't feel the dirty taste and she was proven right. She did specify that she could not let her do the chemo drugs herself and would limit her to heparin and saline. From that day on, depending on the comfort level of the attending nurses our girl would inject saline, heparin into herself. Needless to say, she looked quite thrilled every time she pushed them while an indulgent but alert nurse stood next to her, ready to intervene. I found the scene unfolding in front of me surreal, making me think, "Was that really my young teen so delightedly pushing saline into herself!" She had become her own nurse and I took the actual nurse's permission and started clicking random pictures to share with friends. Many of my friends thought that I should be proud of moments like these, but I had no clue why they saddened me.

Back home we were amused as we overheard Lavanya and Ditto giggling on skype with their friends from

Australia, India and Singapore. She related to them instances about people dropping by and invariably coming around to talking about her balding head and the general public fascination over falling hair. While chatting with friends in India they delightedly discussed how they learned French in India, in Australia and in America. Truly children could make us adults learn a few lessons, and am not talking about French. The most hilarious story came from Aditi in Mumbai, whose French teacher was married to a Japanese and she was learning Sanskrit while living in India, all the while thinking it was Hindi!

I had mentioned before that one of the drugs affected the heart muscle and Lavanya had received it during her first therapy in Mumbai, too. Her heart needed monitoring and she was scheduled for an echo test before the chemotherapy. It was an hour-long test and the doctor made her comfortable, asked for her favorite TV show, put that on and made small talk while he got everything ready. He asked her where she lived. On hearing the answer, he smiled and turned to me to enquire exactly where. When he heard, the smile became wider. It so turned out that he grew up in the same neighborhood, his parents still lived there and then the biggest smile followed on discovering that he was an alumnus of the same school as his patient. The funny thing was the doctor was more excited than the patient at this discovery, probably because he had graduated some twenty years ago and she was still a student there. After the one-hour test we were bid adieu with the sentence, "Hope to see you walking around in the neighborhood." Yes, I hoped, too, that the day was not far when she could join us for the walks around the beautiful neighborhood. I realized that one had to be an adult to get that warm mushy feeling when an unknown neighborhood boy from the same school did well because strangely while Lavanya didn't share my feelings, my friends echoed my thoughts.

The doctors were unbelievably thoughtful and co-operative, as a matter of fact, who was not! These amazing people surrounded us, whether at school, neighborhood or hospital. Lavanya mentioned that she didn't want to miss school every time there was blood draw and chemo. They looked up their schedule, the clinic timings and other aspects to try to book her in for her next chemo after school. She might need to leave 5-10 minutes before school ended, but she wouldn't miss an entire day. I thanked God and them as I wondered how many patients would prefer to adhere to a schedule of school followed by chemotherapy with plans of pursuing homework thereafter. We sent another silent prayer to the Almighty, with the belief, 'If she can, so she will.' Namrata at once corrected me to say, "No ifs Sohini, she can and she will."

The steroid was making her bloated and we had this feeling that our girl was completely exhausted. The continuous ache seemed to be wringing her body of all energy. We were told that the steroids caused more pain during withdrawal but the pain she was undergoing seemed to be breaking her apart. In addition to all this her skin had started bleeding from the stretch marks that had become acutely tender. Her stomach, thighs, shoulders and arms had king sized stretch marks of different colors from dark red, dark purple, blue to light pink depending on the stage they were in. Even the lightest of cotton seemed like sandpaper to her traumatized skin. She moved from one bed to another in the house, trying all the rooms, all positions to get comfortable, to be pain free.

She had fallen in love with the big master bedroom and with the 16th birthday approaching in less than a month she didn't wish for anything to be bought. She just said, "Oh, Mommy, just give me the master bedroom as my 16th birthday present." Huh!!! Actually she had a very worthy winsome argument to support her request. According to her, "You just sleep in your bedroom, you go there at night to sleep and then once out, you don't return to it the whole day. When your friends visit you either sit in the living room, family room or even at the kitchen table. For me, I spend whole night in the bedroom, most days, too, I study in my bedroom, when my friends visit we sit and eat in my bedroom! So who deserves the bigger master bedroom?"

The pain and lethargy were keeping her much in bed, without conversation, no wise cracks, just nothing. Colleges had begun visiting the school giving presentations and she had signed up for a few of them. We attempted the University of California, Berkeley presentation but turned back in less than 10 minutes, as she couldn't sit any longer. There was college fair one evening in the school district and Lavanya was very keen to attend that. We were not in a hurry, but she had this huge enthusiasm and interest to feel and experience the admission atmosphere and process, but we reminded her again that there was a lot of time as she was just a junior. So long she concentrated on getting well, talked to her body to take the therapy as it was supposed to without disrupting her life and health she would get there sooner than later. She stared at me and said, "Mum, I know but I still want to go and am talking to my body but it does not listen anymore." My heart went out to her for her innocent reply, and I could just say, not to worry, I was talking to it, too, and it had to listen to the mother. I also said that I was going to put up an update and tell everyone to send messages to her body, take the chemo, kill the leukemia cells, recuperate, relax, rejuvenate. Varun, though, found 'talking to the body' a little out of his field and limited his talks to us humans rather than the cells and parts of the body.

One day I bumped into an acquaintance who is a psychiatrist. She was concerned whether I had 'anyone to talk to.' I told her yes, I had my best friend. She was surprised as to how I had a 'best friend' in just a year in the States and with due respects, her expression was comical when she realized that I meant my husband as my best friend. I assured her that he, my new friends here, my school friends from three decades ago and the friends I have in Mumbai, Melbourne, Singapore or Germany were all my support. Was I blessed! That was an understatement of the century.

Chapter 31

"Health is a state of complete physical,
mental and social well-being,
and not merely the absence of disease or infirmity."
World Health Organization

When the nurses saw Lavanya turning up for two consecutive chemo appointments in a wheel chair their antenna went up. It was definitely unlike the Lavanya they knew and treated regularly. Our scheduled appointment was adhered to; in the sense we were taken into the fast pod for chemo but thereafter it was held off to have a good proper long look at her. Look good they did! Right from the top of her new sprouting hair to the tip of her purple painted toenails. The conclusion was that she has reacted very aggressively to the previous week's chemo. Some big words that didn't make sense to me were discussed and since she had begun seeing black random spots, the ophthalmologist at Stanford was summoned. To the oncologist, the eyes seemed okay but they wished for the specialist to confirm. The big words meant that her nerves were affected and she was having neurotic pains all over. That was the reason why she hadn't been able to move the entire week. Her feet were cramping and so were the calves, which were a known common side effect, but when the arms, too, cramped up it was unbearably painful. One day as I dried her after bath, her wrist turned as she cramped up. At that time, she did wail with the pain as I physically turned the wrist around, straightened the fingers and massaged it back to position. Later she giggled that it looked straight out of a horror movie or a wicked witch's hands but her comparisons failed to make me laugh.

An MRI was ordered to find the cause of the continuous pain in her back, legs and other joints. The result had us shaken. It revealed that the steroids with chemo had affected her bones making our 17-year-old probably the youngest female with dead bones. Her femur, patella, tibia and fibula were all affected by avascular necrosis that to us laymen meant that her bones had died due to lack of blood supply. She was advised against any high impact activity, as those could lead to small breaks or even collapse of the bones. The short walks on the treadmill that she had begun were stopped immediately and I thought that from then on the only way she could lose the excess weight that had piled on due to the steroids was by way of diet and eventually swimming when the counts were up. And then it stuck me that how could she diet when she was nauseous most of the time! We were in a never ending vicious circle of one issue leading to another.

I knew with all magicians at work our girl would get better but the turnaround was so sudden that it did feel like magic. At dawn she left the bed without groaning, by afternoon she was walking almost normal and by evening planning to go to school within twenty-four hours. The night was peaceful without her calling out to us for either medication or massage. We were in mood for celebration. When one's child moved after almost two weeks, it gave all the reasons in the world to celebrate. I sent messages to our friends that wherever they were and whatever the local time was, they could drink to the magic they created. They could drink anything suitable at that time; drink whatever brought them joy – be it wine, beer, scotch, tea, coffee or even plain H_2O. Shilpi bought a bottle of Moscato to toast from Singapore. Joel and Deepak cheered with their morning tea in Mumbai office and our friends in the States cheered with wine.

When we next went to hospital the nurses were thrilled to see Lavanya walking in rather than the wheel chair ride she had during the previous two appointments. It was heartwarming to see the nurses, their assistants, appointment setters and all those involved in making the whole daunting process work smoothly, sharing every little joy and standing by during those setbacks. We all were both surprised and delighted when she took out French homework to catch up on the two weeks of missed school as we waited for the blood draw results. It was time for most schools to have their homecoming dance and the nurses discussed their respective children's excitement over it. Mine, too, wished to go for her school's homecoming dance and I prayed and wished that she would be well enough to enjoy it.

With great pleasure I shared a picture of Lavanya in all red, set for her homecoming dance. Red defined her attire that evening, with dress, scarf, lips all red, and a natural blush coloring her cheeks. She could stay at the dance for a full thirty minutes! I wondered who was more delighted, she herself, her friends, we or our friends. Waiting in the car to pick up, I saw her friends and her talking to school security as he wondered why that group of girls was leaving early. On hearing from one of her friends that the girl in the red scarf with stars glittering on it covering her head had a chemo the previous day, he looked stumped. Lavanya was blessed to have those friends who left the dance with her to catch a quick dinner together and go home. I thanked them all, Yana, Hikari and Ipek for giving her love and support. The unanimous verdict of 'super friends for a super girl' came pouring in. Not too many could claim to know teens who would leave home-coming dance to be with their friend who wasn't well enough to attend the entire event. Mary Jane felt, "That it was incredible that she was up to it at all. It was a credit to Lavanya's friends that they showed such understanding and support at such a young age. They seem to have maturity beyond their years and their parents and families should be so proud of them." I agreed with her.

At times like this I wondered why there are wars and issues between countries when the children of different nationalities could be great friends, why couldn't nations of educated highly capable adults follow suit! Yana a Russian, Hikari a Japanese, Ipek a Turkish, Amanda a Chinese, Arij a Pakistani and Lavanya an Indian were great friends in California, America. Lavanya always laughed when she related stories of the girls going out. Amanda was the only one who was born and raised in the States while all the others were a year old in the country like us. When walking, they all walked on the left while Amanda pushed them on the right. Getting on escalators they would all go to stand at the one on the left while Amanda would pull them away from the escalators which was coming up and take them towards the right to the escalator that was going down. She with infinite patience taught them about the dime, nickel and quarter in the currency while the girls giggled in confusion. Aussie coins were simple without the dimes and nickels and they had different shapes and sizes to distinguish just by touch. For the longest time even I would push my coin changes to the person at the coffee shop requesting her to take whatever was needed.

We were happy when she went back to baby-sitting the neighborhood twins aged six. On her first visit back they welcomed her joyously – "Lavanya, you are back!! Where did your hair go? Next time bring them also with you!" Oh the innocence of childhood is simply adorable. Lavanya encountered a firsthand experience of individuality and how two kids born a few minutes apart to the same parents could be of contrasting personalities. While one loved board games, the other loved the outdoors. I think she finally appreciated the difference of personality between Ditto and her, understanding his aversion to hours of monopoly over throwing the ball, but of course I wouldn't ask her to admit the same.

Our friends were delighted with all things positive and shared they, too, had begun to appreciate every small thing. Likewise, we made a celebration out of nothing. Life itself is a huge celebration and I realized that we needed to acknowledge that simple but elusive fact every day. Making something out of nothing, taking joys in catnaps, short walks, fragrance of flowers, sounds of birds, a neighbor waving or even an unexpected knock on the door or an impromptu visit by a friend!

Chapter 32

"The more you praise and celebrate your life, the more there is in life to celebrate."

Oprah Winfrey

Despite knowing the highs and the lows of the treatment it was difficult to fathom the lows, go through them, see what they did and for our girl to endure them. One day would be great, with her attending school, baking cupcakes, finishing homework and the next would have her crying with pain and nausea unable to move from the bed. Despite knowing what each medication's side effect was, we were hit hard when the episodes of pain or nausea actually happened and it was an agony to watch her eyes ridden with tears, rolling down her face as she tried hard to find a comfortable painless position to rest. On the bad days when I would peep into Lavanya's room, she would look at me with big doleful eyes and say, "Aw, no school, Mommy? I want to go, I need to go, I don't want to get into the vicious cycle of always catching up."

I also found it strange how families worked, dad couldn't sleep in Mumbai, mum and daughter couldn't in Cupertino and the son in his sleep chattered through the night. Namrata promised to drop by at the earliest to massage and give reiki and Mali brought three different styled wigs that she received as a woman undergoing breast cancer treatment. We did our own little fashion show with longhaired wig, pixie wig and a shoulder-length hair wig. I say we looked cute!

Ditto turned 12 amidst lot of joy, wishes, cake, fun, friends and love. Wishes poured in from everywhere. He had requested for a party at Santa Clara Paintball and that was what was arranged for him and his group of 10 boys. The novice mum had thought Paintball was something to do with painting balls! The cake Lavanya baked for her brother's 12th was beautiful and delicious. It was sheer determination and strength of mind that got her there else she had been pretty much in bed moaning and groaning. My two rocks Mali and Namrata were the major source of support, Mali stayed with Lavanya while I took Ditto to celebrate his birthday with his friends at Santa Clara Paint Ball and Laser tag. Namrata gave me the much needed and appreciated support and company amidst the kids as Varun was overseas. Achala warmed our heart by penning a poem for our boy. Achala became the in-house poetess writing poetry for his birthday followed by one for Lavanya's. I never knew that a dentist could be a great poet too! All the hidden, unknown talents of our friends began blossoming as they tapped into their internal resources to bring happiness.

Lavanya had a long day at hospital with therapy having such complicated sounding drugs- cyclophosphamide, cytarabine, methotrexate and hydrocortisone. I really wondered again as to how the drugs got their names. I complimented the management of the hospital on their efforts in reducing waiting time for procedures and was surprised at their delight on being told that. I realized that we all do complain when things don't work out or are delayed, but when things go right we seldom remember to take the time to appreciate the efforts leading to those improvements. Fortunately, I had been reminding myself to do that all week and I was happy that I could finally tell them, and it looked as though I had made their day. I admit I have reached a stage that I put reminders on the phone for many unthinkable things, which normally I would have remembered simply without a phone beeping reminder. I thought I was bad until the day I heard the better half's phone beeping a reminder – 'Sohini's anniversary.' Oh boy that did it! The fun I had giving him much grief over his own wedding anniversary reminder and that too one that read as Sohini's anniversary. Er ahem, honey what was it to you again?

Namrata shared that her sons were wondering as to how mum turned up every day either with cupcakes, muffins, idli (rice cakes) or some delicacy or the other. I blamed the very Indian mentality of deriving joy from feeding people. If you go to an Indian's home feeling low, you would at once be offered a seat while the host/hostess would cook up some pakoda/chai (fritters/tea) for you. If you go to celebrate something in an Indian's home, you would be presented with an array of sweets and savory. Indians celebrated with food at birth of baby in the family-yes you would find a box of sweets kept conspicuously in the hospital room table. They offered food at the time of death, to deal with sorrow. Be it weddings, funerals, parties or plain and simple visiting each other, food plays a huge role in the Indian culture. Was it any wonder that Namrata was getting sunk with food from all possible direction? For Indians, food was just an expression of love.

Soon it was Lavanya's birthday and Aditi sent a book from India to honor our girl on her 16th. It spoke about the 16 things to love about Lavanya. It gave 16 colorful pages filled with verse, occasions remembered, pictures of times gone by, pictures of aspirations and all things the girls treasure, compiled, written and made with lots of love for the milestone birthday.

A card from Namrata and Mali said, "Life isn't about waiting for the storm to pass; it is about learning how to dance in the rain." Namrata added, "You have taught us all to dance in the rain. I would have wished your life to be filled with sunny bright light but you do not need it, for you are the light yourself. You fill up every heart near you with warmth better than the sun."

Chapter 33

For the visit to hospital following the 16th birthday, Lavanya painstakingly baked two large cakes and 24 cupcakes for all the wonderful people who took care of her. Ditto was delegated with the work of adding sprinkles to the icing. Then, off we went for chemo armed with cupcakes and more cakes for the wonderful doctors, nurses, receptionist and staff who had become such huge parts of our lives that we knew their birthdays, their kid's birthday and what they did on weekends, their favorite food, recipes etc.

The cakes vanished in no time and as we waited for the procedure, thank yous and wishes poured in. When the anesthetist came to her for a chat prior to the procedure, she recognized him as the one who was her anesthetist earlier during port placement surgery. On hearing about the taste of medications bothering her, at the time of the procedure he told her to push the anesthesia into her port and she wondered what if she fell asleep while doing it! He assured her he would take care. Probably with 1/3rd of the medication into her, she said she was sleepy enough for him to take over. I just stood there marveling that our girl graduated from pushing heparin and saline to pushing anesthesia. I appreciated that the doctors prioritized patient safety, comfort and procedure compliance before delegating the responsibility, all the while alert and watchful. What thoughtful ways the doctors and nurses went out of their way to make a child feel comfortable, safe and taken care of. One nurse reminded another to get lots of hot blankets, as Lavanya felt cold on waking up from anesthesia. Another point for appreciation for remembering these small things that matter, amidst the hundreds of patients who are under their care.

When she went into recovery room her primary oncologists Dr Lacayo and others came by and chatted about the soon to begin next phase. Everything from birthday party, PSAT, IB programs, AP courses, chemo fog, Twilight, werewolves, witches, patient preferences and of course the medications were discussed at leisure. Dr Dahl, a lovely gentleman came in smiling, patting his almost concave tummy and saying, "Do you see the difference the cupcake made!"

Lavanya couldn't go to school the entire week after the spinal chemo. It was expected that her counts would drop to lowest of lows as they had before with daily chemo and she would need blood or platelet transfusion. With three years of leukemia treatment in early 2000s and almost 7 months into our present episode, despite no medical background we could read the blood works. I could foresee that the next time's labs would show low ANC as it is a percentage of neutrophils against WBC and the result was as expected. But God is great and I guess we had reached a comfort level with the doctors, nurses and the team because we were let go as we were considered 'responsible parents!' While we all believe ourselves to be responsible parent/spouse/person and try to do things right it was both comforting and amusing to hear it from the medical team. We hurried home lest someone changed their mind about our responsibility levels and made us guests at the oncology floor. A sight to behold was Lavanya trying to merge with the carpet and the wall as she hobbled to the exit before that change of mind occurred.

So we stayed on high alert, checking temperature, watching energy levels, consciously noting all the sounds, coughs and sneezes and their frequency. I thought that we were clearly getting on her nerves as we kept feeling her forehead. Since my hands are always freezing I check my family's temperature by putting my cheeks on their forehead, kind of cumbersome if and when done frequently. Imagine me walking by Lavanya, and every time quickly swinging in to feel her forehead with my cheek! It was a different ball game altogether when you were repeatedly told by everyone that your child was going to fall sick and you were to wait for it to happen, hoping and praying that it didn't!

We knew from experience that one hospitalization turned the entire family, household upside down and of course it was worst for her as she was hooked onto IV, monitors just waiting for the counts to go up, hating the thought of missing school. Kids though manage to find entertainment in the most unlikely places. I recalled I had wondered why she would quietly stare at the monitor and her reply of, "I am watching myself breathe," had left me non-plussed. She would breathe deeply and the pink line would move up and down rhythmically, then she would pant and do shallow breathing to make the pink line go crazy jumping up and dipping down. Fortunately, the nurses were adept at kids doing all kinds of things to keep themselves occupied and this was another prank added to their long list. We continued to have eventless days, slightly cold, little rain, with a chill in the air. While Ditto did homework and Varun worked, Lavanya and I thought of playing UNO and I saw her walking out of Ditto's room giggling and swaying. I didn't think much of it until she said, "Hey, mommy, between his room and the bathroom I banged into the wall six times." A little concerned I wondered why, but she said she was okay, just felt as if she had been sedated before blood transfusion.

We distributed the cards for a game of UNO, but she couldn't move her hand to pick them up. By then she was slightly tearful and scared saying, "This is not funny anymore. What's happening to me? Please put me to bed!" But before I could help her to her room her right leg turned at an angle as she fell and luckily I caught her. I called out to Varun; he stopped work and sat her down on the sofa. He checked her blood sugar first, which was fine, temperature too was normal. She giggled a little as she saw both of us watching her constantly, but again that giggle turned to a sob as she felt her tongue swelling up and when her speech slurred we made the SOS call to the afterhours oncologist on call.

As we waited for the call back, my phone lit up with a message from Shilpi, just asking her usual query as to how things were. I replied, giving status update and she in turn informed Usha, Jayshree, her Buddhist chanting group and others. Namrata sent a message giving a recipe I had requested for and I updated her, too. Everyone started a collective prayer session in different parts of the world. Soon almost like magic, Lavanya's inexplicable strange symptoms were reducing, some feeling returned to the right side of her body, speech became normal, too. I would like to believe it was the power of prayers that eased the symptoms as miraculously as they had appeared and within an hour or so she was almost normal except for the walking.

I might be biased but when Lavanya sighed, "Please tell the aunties to fix my head, too, as it feels numb with pain," I knew that my girl, too, was touched by the prayers and wishes. She felt delighted when she could lift her right hand without support from her left hand and with Varun's help managed to go to her room. The night was that of vigil with Varun and me taking turns to watch her and help her to the rest room. We headed for the hospital first thing in morning to investigate the reason for the previous night's scary episode.

One of our favorite nurse practitioners, Jen Owens met us immediately and did all kinds of tests to check on neurological functions. As Dr Lacayo was not available, she brought in another doctor with 30 years' experience in leukemia/lymphoma. He did similar tests as Jen. She was asked to push his hands hard and everyone had a good laugh when he staggered under the force. He wisely and sportingly took precautions of moving aside when he checked her leg strength. Good for him because that too was found fine and strong. Verdict was that it was the spinal tap of the previous week that seemed to have momentarily affected the side of her brain responsible for controlling the motor movements and speech.

Poulomi warmed my heart when she wrote in that she couldn't believe that amidst all that was on, our girl phoned Aditi to wish her happy birthday. I do love these childhood friendships where nothing, not even left part of the brain not working properly stops a person from thinking of a special friend.

Why certain reactions happened to some kids, when it happened or the duration of it was difficult to predict or even understand, so another meeting with the primary oncologist to figure out the next course of action was scheduled. He, meanwhile was talking to other leukemia specialists around the country. Pre meds, post meds, drug monitoring, drug combo, everything was done for her when the drug methotrexate was given as that was what was suspected to have caused that seizure in May. There were seven more spinal taps and plenty more methotrexate remaining over next two years. She was advised no school until the counts came up. I told everyone to keep praying as believing them was feeling them and the feeling was good. We went back home, Varun working in office, me working in kitchen and Lavanya catching up on sleep. The only person in the family to continue normal day-to-day life, Ditto was in school and I was glad that he was able to continue his routines amidst all that was going on. One day he asked me, "Mummy, so how long since the diagnosis and treatment, two years?" He couldn't it believe when I said seven months, because it did feel like forever. It is ironical how fast good times pass whereas how difficult it was to tide over difficult time.

In Christine's words, "Oh Sohini to watch your child in pain has and will always be more painful than enduring one's own pain. I know you are stronger and have a resolve that is greater than anyone else I have ever seen, but reading this post and thinking what can I do to share what you are going through and somehow dilute it to make it more bearable leads me to believe as humans we are incredibly powerful. If we believe we are able to lighten your load by all together sharing the pain and in doing so allow us all to share in prayer, then I know that with each incident there will be hope that together we shift its direction back to where it needs to go. So, Lavanya, will endure and come through at the end of treatment unbeaten! Stay strong dear friend."

Chapter 34

"All the world is full of suffering.
It is also full of overcoming."

Helen Keller

The mother who cried time!! That was my new name. Just as in the folklore the boy who cried wolf, I had been re-christened the mother who cried time. Apparently at 6.00 a.m. I would wake the kids up saying that it was 6.15, if the appointment at the hospital was at 10.00, I would say it was at 9.30 and so on. Always playing with time to be on time but I found it funny that in all their awareness of the same the kids humored me. But the fun was on me when I realized that they played the same game with me. If Lavanya needed to be at school at 9.00 she would tell me 8.50, again keeping that extra time for her to walk slowly to her class.

Life was looking sunnier for Lavanya with counts on an upward swing, pain diminishing to negligible levels and ability to attend school more frequently. The most relieving part for her was that mum didn't turn up every so often putting her cheek against her forehead to check temperature. I think mums and dads could beat any thermometer hollow for checking their child's temperature, and we didn't even have to go under the armpit or inside the mouth! Thank God for that! We know their normal temperature so well that we could just hold onto them to know if it was not normal. We spent lot of time simply chatting, reading, cooking or baking. I was mixing the cake batter for an upside down cake while Lavanya caught her breath from the job and suddenly smiled, "Hey, Mommy, why do we say upside down? Why not downside up?" Before I could even think of an answer, she pondered further, "Why is it inside out and not outside in?" Staying home and doing random things brought out interesting queries to which I had no answer and wonder if the savior of all, Google would either.

The Indian festival of lights Diwali, a celebration of the good over evil, too, was to be celebrated over the weekend and we lit diyas (candles) in and around the house with prayers. I also like to believe that it was the triumph of good cells over the leukemia cells, the rise of the hemoglobin and WBC and all things nice. We spent a good amount of time indoors watching the magic of Tom Hanks and I realized that he is the one actor whose movies could be watched with family, where mum, dad and kids could all sit together and enjoy nice feel good movies. We watched movies we had watched before and caught up again with kids, – *Apollo 13* and *Catch me if you can,* were fantastic. Later we went out to watch a Bollywood movie. Varun, Lavanya and I had to desperately smother our giggles as everyone including our Ditto very quietly watched an intense scene.

The scene I write about was that of the wheel chair bound villain finding a compatible bone marrow from a virtuous person, transfers it into his body using huge pipes (San Jose water company could be put to shame with those pipes), sounds and special effects so much so that at the end of the procedure, the virtuous person was in a wheel chair while the villain was able to walk, run and jump around to spread tyranny. Hilarious to the point of being hysterical.

But no, I wished moviemakers would be more sensible as well as responsible when making these movies. No wonder with a population of over a billion in India bone marrow donors are far and few. I had to at once tell Ditto that this was NOT what actually happens. Poor kid, what must be going on in his mind because earlier there was a discussion about bone marrow transplants with him as the donor.

The last few months had made us realize that stem cell transplant and bone marrow transplant were simple procedures, just like blood transfusion requiring a compatible donor and then lo and behold just a thing in the bag getting into your body. No lights, camera, action, pipes absolutely nothing, zilch! It was the before and after care and treatment that were draining and time consuming. I wished that this knowledge was more widespread and commonly known to everyone, especially in Asian communities and countries to facilitate donors to volunteer and register themselves as the registry is sorely lacking in Asian donors.

Lavanya had been thinking of fund-raising next summer for donating to research for finding that one pill cure to leukemia. She had been making soaps, cards and cupcakes to pass the time when counts were low. Achala shared a URL which touched us and made all of us smile. It was the same 'Make a Wish Foundation' which was going to make Lavanya's wish, too, come true. Make a Wish Foundation turned San Francisco into Gotham city so a five-year-old leukemia patient's wish of meeting batman could be made true. They went those many extra steps to coordinate and organize so that the kid was Batkid, the savior of Gotham city and the city mayor even presented him with the keys to the city. Volunteers became onlookers, robbers, getaway car drivers to complete the show, as bat kid in training with batman saved a city. The same Make a Wish Foundation made Lavanya's wish of visiting Paris come true after the end of her treatment. It came complete with a stretch limo pick up that had napkins the color of French flags, a sealed envelope for the flight crew who welcomed Ms. Lavanya Rajpal specifically on the flight and the captain invited her with the brother in tow for a visit to the cockpit with an announcement welcoming her to Paris. So many thoughtfully planned events, big or small, made a huge difference to the child battling the disease, as she felt honored, loved and special along with her family.

Mary Jane and Marion both researched methotrexate extensively and felt it had a lot to answer for. And I thought how sweet it was that they found the will and time to read about the medication their friend's daughter was taking!

And they were not the only ones. There were many friends who between themselves, their spouse and kids had done so much reading and research on leukemia that most were well informed on drug toxicity, effects and side effects. That set me wondering what was methotrexate. On looking up on the Internet I realized this drug was synthesized by an Indian biochemist and then clinically developed by an American pediatrician. It was on the WHO list of Essential Medicines required in a basic health system and it was only in 1947 that its use in treatment of acute lymphoblastic leukemia was seen. Pretty noteworthy was that despite being around for that long, its side effects and toxicity were not fully understood neither could they be forecast.

After months of treatment we had learned to take good news with great celebration and nasty surprises with calmness. So when during regular labs for some strange reason saline could be pushed into her port but no blood draw was possible, we didn't get concerned. Lavanya did some acrobatics, moved her arms up and around and after three syringes of saline emptied into her, we were gifted with a trickle of blood that steadily became normal and blood draw was successful. We didn't have to wait for reports so we were in and out in less than 30 minutes. There was a repeat the next day of the same again. The nurses could push saline into her port but not get blood in the line. What was up with Lavanya! All the acrobatics were repeated without luck. Except for standing upside down, er sorry downside up, everything was tried. Left arm up, right hand down, right hand up, left hand down, both hands up, both down, lying on back, turning on each side but no, the blood was elusive. While the input was happening with saline going in, the output was zero with no blood coming out! No blood draw meant, no chemo. The doctor said if the anesthetist agreed to go through with the anesthesia, the spinal chemo will be on schedule and the anesthetist said if she could push in the meds and fluids she was fine to go ahead. So spinal chemo happened with clockwork precision. Another medicine that unclogs the port was administered thereafter to clear the line for blood draw and the wait of 45 min for it to work its magic began. I was reminded of all the liquids, gels, granules and powders available in supermarkets for clearing clogged/ blocked drains! Similarly, Lavanya's port was getting unclogged with a medical equivalent of the above.

We were still in the recovery room where another child, probably 5-6 years old was wheeled in after his procedure across the curtain. When Lavanya realized that the child was to start Interim Maintenance 1 with high dose methotrexate requiring 3-5 days admitting in another hospital, she got talking to the mum. The mum was delighted to get all the information on the new hospital from a person who had been there and done that. The three Fs that played an important role – Food, fun and friend, where methotrexate was the 'friend' visiting, and fun was the option of numerous hospital activities available. Suddenly the mum looked closely at Lavanya and asked, "Are you the one who would take spinal chemo without anesthesia?" And I thought whoa! Stories did travel.

We realized that 70 percent of the Nurse Practitioners were pregnant and probably a good 75% of nurses were, too. Lavanya wondered what would happen when they all went on maternity leave! I did mention to them that everyone in oncology seemed to be expecting and they laughed, "Sohiniiiii, don't drink the water here!!!" And of course, talk about my big mouth and me! It has a tendency to run away from me. I was sharing the joke about staying away from hospital water with our social worker Kate and she couldn't stop laughing, literally bending at the waist as she continued to laugh and gasped, "Oh Sohiniii! Did I tell you that am pregnant! Yes, you please carry your water bottle."

Many laugh that it didn't take much to touch me, that I was overwhelmed maybe faster than others, more sentimental, a little more emotional. Probably guilty as charged. The other day Lavanya mentioned that she wished to watch a movie, but all her friends refused to watch it with her. The movie, *Fault in Our Stars* based on a book by John Green, was the story of a teen girl with cancer and I could empathize with her friends' wish to not watch it with her. Lavanya couldn't understand why, though I appreciated the thought. But then where there was a will there definitely was a way. Lavanya found her soul mate, fellow cancer victor Tanvi who had become a good friend while hooked onto IV receiving BFF methotrexate in neighboring rooms and these two teenagers undergoing treatment decided to watch *Fault in Our Stars* together. I said to the girls, "Cheers to YOU, your grit, your determination, your will and humor for the treatment you are going through, for life, all things good, bad and ugly that you take in your stride with a wisdom beyond your years and anyone's comprehension." Lavanya's comment, "We could go as the cancer couple, one wearing red and the other wearing white, depicting red blood cells and white blood cells," had us in splits and I kept up with the joke adding, "Take me with you, I will come as platelet."

Aparna commended Lavanya and wondered how tough it must be for the sibling, too. She wondered if all the challenges that we as a family were going through had made our boy grow up at a tender age or not. She felt that every mum would be proud to be the mother of such kids and I agreed. I agreed that they were responsible for my feelings of gratification, strength, love and happiness. I wondered if I felt proud? The dictionary meaning of proud is pleased, glad, happy along with smug, pompous, snobbish and some more unflattering adjectives. As a mum I wouldn't like to draw feelings of smug, pompous, snobbish relating to the beautiful beings that are my children. So, no I am not proud, am just plain and simple happy.

Our children's high school has a particular day; a Thursday in March and November dedicated for talking about challenges students faced and overcame and is called Challenge Day. As I write, it is Challenge Day again and Lavanya told me, "Oh, Mommy, two years back as a Sophomore I shared on Challenge Day Thursday that ten years ago I had cancer and everyone around me was shocked because only a few close friends were aware of the past illness." Surprise of surprises, the Challenge Day of senior year she told them, "Hey, guess what? Two years ago on a Challenge Day Thursday I shared that I had cancer and it came back the following Tuesday and I am still undergoing chemotherapy for it. How bizarre is that!" While she laughed and wondered about this, I quietly listened, with a blank mind and no words.

Chapter 35

"When one is willing and eager, the Gods join in."
Aeschylus

As I worked in the kitchen I kept stealing glances at my girl sitting at the table twirling her short mop of curls staring hard at her laptop screen. What would have been otherwise long straight hair was now a mass of curls giving her face a cuteness that surpassed what the pre chemo long straight hair might have done. She would look at me once in a while with a silent query and go back to staring at the screen. Suddenly she turned to me exasperated as well as agitated asking, "Oh, Mommy! What do I write?" Yes, our cancer victor, not once but twice was trying hard to figure out her personal statement and essay for the University of California freshman admission and few east coast colleges. Past two years while she was struggling with chemotherapy and its side effects, barely able to write because of neuropathic fingers, moving with difficulty due to dead bones, life went on normally for those around her and her peers were all done with their SATs, essays and college applications, and she was only beginning. With one month to college applications, a week for SATs and God knows how many essays to write she was suitably concerned. As a mum my heart broke thinking of her wish to excel against all odds, though Varun suggested that she needed to do only what she could without stress. We were happy for her to take a break, to continue after full recovery or she could attend the very good community colleges in the neighborhood transferring to a college once the treatment was over and she regained a regular healthy life.

She was a student of a school of very ambitious, high achievers who worked on a string of activities to add to their resume, many preferring quantities over quality. There was always a race to accomplish the utmost in the least time. Parents dedicated their lives driving the kids from piano/flute to SAT class to Advanced Placement tuition followed by a quick dinner probably in a parking lot. I saw kids taking life so seriously that I shuddered to think what would happen when they grew up and life really happened.

As an onlooker I felt that on one hand there were these highly stressed students working on every possible aspect and on the other it appeared as though colleges were looking for a rock climber who was a first class rower with exceptional debating skills. Someone who worked with the underprivileged, traveled around the world volunteering time and effort combined with a SAT score of over ninety percent, a simple 4.0 GPA (Grade Point Average) and could portray their skills in a way that could only be called humble bragging. With the world embracing self-promotion, humility would soon be restrained to history and dictionary. And here was our girl, the other extreme, who didn't consider herself proficient in one particular field though I felt she was undermining herself. To most she seemed to be a sum total of all things positive, a girl focused on every little thing that she did and she did them well. She seemed to be one of those rare few who studied because of love of the course, subject and not for the college credits it would entail. However, she personally, was drawing a blank. In today's world self-propaganda and self-promotion are the expected and accepted norms and she was a quiet, humble misfit. On hearing me call her humble, her newly grown eyebrows shot up as she giggled, "Me and humble!"

I looked at my agitated teen and suggested that she could talk about herself and I was not the only one suggesting that. I had heard that aspiring college applicants needed to tell their story and I reminded her what many had said to her, "Girl, you have one hell of a story." Tell the story. Her story didn't have all the factors that she would have pursued under normal circumstances helping make that sought after resume but it did encompass a whole lot more that was achieved under unusually difficult circumstances, that unfortunately could not be part of any resume. Life's lessons do not give any Degree, Diploma or Certificate. They just mold and shape the personality for achieving that perfect balance with a stability of dedication and a softness of empathy. I am not too sure whether she wrote anything about her story as she didn't share her essays with us thinking we would be biased and applaud blindly. Would we? Yes, we would applaud definitely, but biased, I don't think so. I believed that what was visible was very apparent and transparent. I saw that she worked hard and achieved great results. How many children manage to work hard, diligently through their high school years undergoing treatment for blood cancer maintaining a positive outlook?

My belief that when God brings you to it, he will lead you through it, was proven right yet again when her wish to do well combined with perseverance and hard work saw her acing all tests with a mind blowing SAT score of 98% altogether, with 100% in Writing and Math! This coupled with a high GPA opened doors to many of her dream colleges and she was in that enviable position to choose from her wish list. If I come across as the 'least' humble bragger, do excuse me, as that definitely is not the intention. The idea is to cite the example to prove that when one is willing and eager, nothing can hinder the path to happiness and success, not even cancer and all the paraphernalia that comes as a package deal with it.

We live in an era that has an information overload, usually very useful but at times scary and overwhelming. We live in times when there are lot of talkers but few listeners, more writers but few readers. Research shows that every three minutes a person is diagnosed with blood cancer in the United States itself. It is also a fact that in children leukemia is one of the most common cancers with one in three cases. I looked at my daughter and told myself this, too, will pass just as it had before. We just had to continue treating it as we did before, treat it with love in the form of chemotherapy so the medicines worked, passing through her body, killing the cancerous cells, with her emerging cured, just waiting to write an exciting story, not of a disease but of her achievement. Of her not being a cancer survivor but a crusader, a true victor.

Unfortunately, no exact cause for leukemia has been discovered so far. When the cause is known for an effect, one can avoid the cause, but when the cause is unknown one can go on exploring, researching and developing new theories and drugs to ultimately reach a cure. In January 2015 there was a controversial article that stated that apart from all the scientific reasons known to cause cancer a part of it was just plain and simple bad luck. Last half a century it has been said that most cancers are caused by mutations either inherited or caused by environmental factors. I have no medical background and I don't know whether the cause is mutation, environmental factors or simply bad luck. All I know is what I have seen from where I have stood – at my daughter's bedside, as a very helpless mother. I have seen what this mutation or the bad luck can do. Having seen firsthand what the disease is, its sheer capabilities and the marathon difficult treatment it entails I tried to bring more light to this dark disease, not scientifically but as a mum. Scientists, doctors and researchers have immense knowledge and are continuing their crusade against the disease but as a mum my knowledge was pretty much zero, I knew nothing. My family had no clue. We learned with diagnosis, we grasped a lot more with treatment and with a step closer to a cure today we have evolved. I have immense respect and deep gratitude for all the scientists and doctors who are dedicated in researching for a cure and developing new therapies. However, there is one therapy that probably doesn't get highlighted enough and that is the therapy of hope, love, prayers, positivity and belief. Combined with drugs and treatment these factors make one unbeatable combination.

Chapter 36

"When it rains look for rainbows,
when it's dark look for stars."

Unknown

As we neared the end of intense therapy I realized that we had applied the above quotation in our lives. By looking at the pluses every day and learning from the minuses, we had strengthened ourselves. The year also saw our boy getting into the Cupertino National Little League and he replaced his cricket bat with a baseball bat. It was fun hearing one of the player's dad say, "Oh so he played ball with a bat that looks like a paddle?" and I laughed, "Yep, and he now plays ball with a bat that resembles a club." Boys are simple – give them a ball and a bat, irrespective of the size and shape, they would connect, building friendships alongside. He loved the game and was awarded Rookie of the Year at the end of the season where his team won the championship. So I learned a little about the home runs, home stretch terminology of baseball and could use it in life. We were definitely on the home stretch of our treatment.

The next stage of treatment Interim Maintenance 2 brought nausea while up and aches when lying down. Lavanya was so drained and tired that she couldn't eat due to zero appetite or dress/undress on her own due to weakness. It was heart wrenching to literally hear the effort she had to make while sipping water, as if every breath was a marathon. Every loud painful sip that I heard squeezed my heart a little more. A low-grade fever set in and we monitored through the night to see if it reached the level when the oncologist on call had to be phoned. As always the first half of the night was my vigil and the second half was Varun's. Marriages are truly made in heaven else how does one explain this perfect partnership where I could stay up late and he could wake up at unearthly hours with both having difficulty in doing what the other accomplished easily. To cut a long night short I was woken up with the news of fever at 102, that call to oncology made and as expected were immediately summoned to ER.

Stanford introduced this little blue card for its onco kids that said, "I am immuno-compromised and need immediate attention at ER." It gave details of allergies, port access procedure, needle size, etc., with contact details of Stanford doctor treating the child. So anywhere in the nation if their onco kid needed attention, instructions were made available for the ER doctors, nurses and staff. When their review system called to check whether the new cards were effective, I had happily told them that while we were very appreciative of the initiative, we had fortunately not had to put it to test. I had optimistically thought of unpacking my hospital overnighter as I had assumed that our days of sudden admitting/ER visits were history, but Varun had said to let it be. And lo and behold we were off again, overnighter in the boot driving to ER.

I intended to call the review team to let them know that the blue card worked like a dream in Stanford ER. We had the benefit of the oncologist on call giving prior intimation to the ER staff of our imminent arrival but still I would say it was an experience without a single hiccup just as it was intended. Despite being in immense pain and discomfort even our ever-critical teen remarked, "Hey, Mommy, they have become super-efficient!"

As the ER nurse came to access her, Lavanya asked if she could have an onco nurse access her as the previous few times access had been traumatic and painful. They readily agreed and the onco team arrived into ER with their kit and both the teams exclaimed with oohs and aahs at the differences in each other's access kits. Unfortunately, with three attempts there was still no blood in the line but fortunately the onco team realized what the issue was. The culprit were the scar tissues that had made her port tender and while it could take the saline, the needle was not long enough to get the blood drawn through all tissues. Thereafter, Lavanya graduated to a one and half inch needle from a one-inch needle for port access until the scar tissues healed. They planned to check if one and quarter inch needles were available because the one and half inch needle stuck out of her dangerously. Blood draw showed that her hemoglobin was at a very low level, requiring transfusion. We went back to One North, the onco floor for a short stay for the transfusion that eventually got over past 9 p.m. The boys welcomed us back as if we had been gone for months and not just 16 hours.

It was Thanksgiving in America, though probably the world, too, celebrates and believes in this beautiful occasion now. What a lovely thought to thank and appreciate all the little things as well as the big ones. While one begins by thanking God for all things bright and beautiful, feeling grateful to those in our lives was a warm feeling because it showed that our lives were full and enriched by their presence.

Our list for thanking was endless. I was blessed to be able to share that we have lovely long list of family and friends who had touched us in one way or the other. So I requested everyone to accept a collective huge grateful thank you. It had been a smooth week with no hospital runs, no aches, pains or any major issue. I went grocery shopping and at the checkout counter the cashier smiled remarking that I looked happy and I replied that actually I was. It had been a nice long weekend and the kids were back at school. She agreed that the breaks were wonderful but when the kids went back to school and routine began, that, too, felt excellent. A few more shoppers and cashiers joined the conversation to echo similar thoughts. I didn't tell them that for us when both kids were in school, it felt even greater. It was better than excellent – it was normal. I now realize normal is the most undervalued aspect of life and is truly precious. Cancer has taught us to appreciate normal, feel grateful for routine and anticipate each day with gratitude.

Lavanya had been feeling a lot better than before with the therapy spaced out to once in ten days. We had come a long way from the daily IV confined to hospital bed on diagnosis to the current stage of three or four visits a month to the hospital for blood draw and chemo. So our girl wanted to give back, starting with the hospital where she got treated, to the Leukemia and Lymphoma Society (LLS) to help their research for the 'one pill cure' instead of the 36 months of treatment. We wrote to LLS sharing our thoughts and ideas and they called back saying they would like to meet us to take her thought forward. So to start in a small way our girl was turning her love for baking into fund raising. On hearing that Lisa gave the much-needed first push, an introduction by placing the first order – moist chocolate cake with chocolate frosting, for a birthday at her work place. It was starting in a small way but then every little thing did count and all small things added up to make something big.

Very often waiting for lab results and chemo we would pass time chatting with the nurses and those around for caregiving. Sometimes someone would share reviews of a movie or show a few dance steps they learned. A nurse proudly showed jewelry made by her daughter, while Lavanya gave impromptu French tutorial to us. We were enlightened with the knowledge that 'bonne chance' meant good luck, but, of course, none of us got the pronunciation or the accent right. Another nurse showed us pictures of her Aussie sister-in-law cooking turkey in Sacramento and wondered about the Aussie equivalent. We came up with 'Boxing Day' and had to at once put their minds to rest that Boxing Day had no gloved fists or ring involved but presents which were 'boxed' that day, typically the day after Christmas. Actually there are other theories, too, regarding the origin and purpose of Boxing Day prevalent in most English settlements, but the one aspect that affected all in current days was that it was a day of celebration and most importantly a holiday.

While the talks of festivities continued the blood report arrived and we were informed that she had aced the blood test. She had exceptional counts for a full dose chemo and so was advised to continue whatever she was doing the entire week because she had definitely done something right. Lavanya bemoaned that she had done pretty much nothing except study and catch up on homework. The verdict was homework and studies agreed with her blood counts.

As the chemo went on it seemed like all staff present were into reminiscing of days gone by as each one remembered their days in high school, how they studied for SATs or AP exams or if in her shoes they would not think of giving exams by re-scheduling chemotherapy. Yes, that was what she did for full 15 minutes to convince them, the importance of postponing chemo by a few days to avoid chemo fog and pain of lumbar puncture just a day before the exams. We returned home amidst laughs of confusion caused by my statement that this morning temperature was -1 degrees. They grinned, "Honey, where exactly are you coming from!" I spoke in Celsius and they understood Fahrenheit. Just when I was giving myself a pat for getting used to the American way of Gallons, pounds, left hand drive, mm/dd/yy, etc., I realized I could never learn enough.

Alka wrote in with wishes for a lifetime filled with raindrops on roses and whiskers on kittens and verses from the song *'Favorite Things'* from *The sound of music*. I thought about kittens and thought good heavens! Lavanya had better not hear/see anything about kittens. It so happens that she wants a kitten as a pet and our boy wants a dog. We moved multiple times making a pet a difficult family member to have. I have known of pets refused visas to Australia and even America. I had heard of people leaving their pets behind with family and friends to endless feelings of guilt and unhappiness. So, goldfish it was for us! When the kids really insisted I promised them both their pets – as wedding gifts. Ditto would get a dog and Lavanya a cat on their respective wedding days. My grand plans came crashing down when Ditto wondered aloud, "But what if my wife is allergic to dogs!!!" And he had just turned 12, right!

Stanford looked beautiful during Christmas, all decked up with a traditional Christmas tree, music, big red fire engine in the drive-way with a highly impressive Santa, lights, balloons and much more. If one wasn't aware that most of the kids around were battling some serious illness or the other one couldn't have guessed by looking at their happy faces. The hospital entrance could easily have been mistaken for the entrance of Disney Land, all one had to do was overlook the masks, IV poles, wheel chairs and tubes. The place echoed with cries of joy, laughter and softly playing music of jingle bells, Rudolph the red nosed reindeer and other Christmas songs. The children smiled through their pain and sickness while the parents reflected their children's emotions.

Next time we checked in, I heard the receptionist call out, "'Lavanya is here." I overheard someone asking "'Now?" I smiled to myself when the receptionist whispered, "Oh they are always on time so they are not called ahead of schedule." The treatment period was so long that over the months not only did the parents get to know the doctors, nurses, aides and others involved very well, but they, too, gathered a lot about the families thereby giving those who ran perpetually late an earlier than scheduled time, proving that I was not the only one who 'lied' about time to be on time.

The recovery room nurses were gracious hostesses when they offered us chocolates for the season. The chemo nurse soon came in to administer the rest of the IV chemo and told us about her forthcoming wedding for which she and her fiancé were practicing Salsa dancing. All done, we returned home and Varun welcomed us back with freshly squeezed orange/carrot/apple juice. Yeah, some men were plain and simple special. He did so many little things for us that he never had to put his love in words and say I love you. He gave me bed tea on days he knew I was fatigued, tried a heart froth on the morning coffee, too! Ditto at twelve years of age got to ride piggy back to the bathroom every morning from his bed, our girl received freshly squeezed juices, exquisite cuisine on demand. I got emptied dishwasher all mornings and flowers on random days for no occasion at all. Fortunately, Ditto was inculcating all that he saw and I could already see a loving husband and dad over and beyond a sensitive son and loving brother.

27th Dec 2013 was our next Chemo, marking the end of Interim Maintenance 2 and the end of the intense nine months' chemo, graduating to once a month IV chemo and probably twice a month hospital visit. Life was looking better and we hoped to celebrate the New Year with new beginnings, closing a painful chapter as well as end our blog. It had served its purpose of giving regular updates to all concerned, brought our friends and family closer to us, blessed our girl with world-wide prayers, in short it brought us a marvelous revelation through everyone. It showed that all good and great were possible when your family and friends had your back just as all things wonderful were achievable with belief and trust. I told our buddies to watch that space next weekend, 28th Dec 2013 to praise God almighty, to thank everyone collectively for achieving another miracle!

Chapter 37

"Feeling gratitude and not expressing it is like wrapping a present and not giving it."
William Arthur Ward

Our friend's huge yay resonated around the world. Quoting Mary Jane again, "This year has been one 'hell-of-a-time' for all of you and now there is relief from the intensity. You are all remarkable and Lavanya can only be admired for the attitude adopted toward all the discomfort and pain that has come with this illness and its required treatment. It is wonderful to read this post. It's full of hope and all things positive. Thank you for allowing us into your world so that we can be there in spirit. Although we are so far away we can direct our prayers to where they are most needed. Have an amazing Christmas time. Take care of yourselves and I await your post of 28th December." In Priya Devotta's words, "So honored to be here in the blog, thank you for letting me share in your family's journey. I've been inspired, learnt so much & am a better person for it. Wishing you all the best of best, health, happiness & togetherness always & in the New Year." The power of people held us through the most unimaginably difficult time and their prayers had brought us to the summit. Together we had prevailed.

I warned our friends that what was going to follow was to be the Mother of all Oscar speeches and they would need to bear with me. I gave good amount of warning that the last entry in the blog was going to be long. I would not be giving updates thereafter during the 18 to 20 months' maintenance treatment as I had hopes and expectations of it being a smooth sailing. This one was to commemorate new beginnings starting then, Dec 27th 2013. It was to honor people, our family and friends. It also was an effort to express something that was going to be very difficult to express in words or actions. We had prevailed only because of what all our friends and family did, individually and collectively.

On 27th Dec 2013 Lavanya completed the intensive treatment for Acute Lymphoblastic Leukemia that had commenced on diagnosis on 26th March 2013. We had a long way to go with the anticipated treatment end day as July 11th 2015 followed by bone marrow test, lumbar puncture and surgery to remove the port. However, we had come a long way since the diagnosis. This long arduous journey was made possible by the two Ps – the Patient herself and the People we had as family and friends. My family was full of gratitude and wanted to express their thanks to each one who had held our hand, helped with prayers and countless wishes.

Family Ties ...

I started with the patient herself, our girl, Lavanya. What could I say of the girl who on diagnosis wondered if she could take the Chemistry test scheduled the next day, voluntarily opted for no anesthesia for spinal chemotherapy, joked about things none of us would dream joking about, laughed at herself the most while pushing herself beyond boundaries, crying in pain bravely, consistently showing an understanding beyond her age, a resilience we hadn't known or heard of and an iron will to move ahead. Girl, I am blessed to be your mum.

To our boy, if a newborn could smile, this one proved it at birth. He indeed was born smiling, so happy he was to be in this big gorgeous world that he just went on happily, with a great goodness of heart and innocence beyond comprehension, Ditto made everything simple because he was simplicity and goodness himself. The last nine months were not exactly easy for the sibling but we didn't hear one complain, no whines and no fuss. He showed responsibility beyond his 11 years when at the time of crisis, he followed instructions and packed his bag to stay at our friend's and neighbor's homes while Varun and I were needed at the hospital, traveling alone to New Jersey to spend holidays with Lubna and Nafis. Yes, our boy grew up way before time and beautifully so.

I truly believe that nothing can go wrong if you married your best friend. This divine knowledge didn't dawn upon me two decades back when we married, but after the many years behind us, I knew, I had done something right. When life was beautiful even without socializing, parties, shopping or holidays, just sitting at home together, waiting out another difficult episode of chemo to pass, you realized that together you can create magic. To my husband, my best friend at the cost of sounding cliché, I was not myself without him – he made me who I am and even though I say it myself, I am not too bad.

My sister and brother-in-law who under different circumstances would have flown in by the first flight as they had done not once but many times in the past when our kids had fallen sick, Lavanya again with leukemia and Ditto with a malfunctioning kidney for which he underwent partial nephrectomy. This time they lent support with calls and prayers as my dear sister herself was fighting a life-threatening condition to which we lost her in August 2013. My mother-in-law who offered prayers in every temple she could, followed every superstition she would have probably laughed at earlier, but with belief she followed them. She fed the cow, planted saplings, woke up early for a prayer and slept late because of another; she did all that only a grandma could do, quietly and religiously.

The friendly neighborhood ...

Our dear friends – we will forever pray for showers of blessings on them ... Nafis and Lubna for leaving everything and taking the first flight across the nation to be with us on diagnosis and later to help. Our neighbors Srini and Vishnu, Pat and Pauahi, Gina, Leslie, Karen, Dan, Anita, Gary, Bev – I thanked them for keeping their doors open to take in our boy whenever required, the endless prayers at church, visits to the chapel, food, cookies, quilt, fruits and a whole lot of love. We were seven months 'new' in the country and the neighborhood, but thanks to them we never felt like strangers. Jhoomar, my friend from childhood – the first person I sent the message on diagnosis calling, 'help' – she and her family turned up with such rock solid support that we didn't need much thereafter. Gita and Ashwin spoilt us with an endless array of food, games, thoughtful visits, support and Ditto loved the days he spent with them going to Lake Tahoe. All their prayers and chanting touched us to last forever. Mali, another childhood friend whom I discovered at Jollyman Park next door gave us a new lease with her strong support and introduced us to Namrata, another one from our little town Nagpur, who had made her home in the Bay Area. Namrata spent hours healing Lavanya with reiki and acupressure despite her busy schedule. Lisa, Lavanya's chiropractor, friend, philosopher and guide and in turn ours, too – I couldn't count in how many ways she added cheer to our days, reduced pain and helped in more ways than one could think of. Always with a spring in her step, a smile in her eyes, she encouraged all things nice without reservation. Lavanya's friend Yana's regular presence at her hospital bedside boosted not only her, but also the whole family.

Great School Ratings proved right ...

Great School Ratings website brought us to Cupertino as we consciously searched for an 'excellent public school' to transition to from the 'world class private school' our kids attended in Melbourne. The website was right when it gave both the Middle School and High School our kids go to ten out of ten. The website www.greatschools.org was what we had consulted to know more about schools when

269

moving to America and its ratings of ten being the highest from all perspectives was met by both our schools. I felt that the actual numbers deserved to be way over and beyond the given credit. We received something more than just academics or curriculum as the school principal, assistant principal, dean, teachers, staff, students and community rose up to the occasion beyond expectation to provide support. Without their understanding an already tough year would have been tougher. Mrs. Scott, Mr. Hicks, Ms. Onodera, Ms. Finck, Mr. Ruskus, Ms. Bana, Mr. Goldenkranz, Ms. Lomme, Mr. Clark, Mr. Otto, Mr. Kim, Ms. Smith, Ms. Maxwell, Ms. Kruse organized everything for Lavanya, very thoughtfully and methodically, so much so that despite irregular attendance not only was she able to understand the course, but also maintained and nurtured that love for learning. The school color quilt so lovingly made by the students and teachers is going to be cherished forever. Her home schooling teacher Ms. Hershey gave her a freedom of pace to complete all her course within a stipulated time, all the while bridging the gap between school and home school. Mr Matt Wright, the history teacher for home school rekindled Lavanya's love for the subject all over again with his extensive knowledge, enthusiasm and proficiency. I thanked God for pushing us in this direction when we moved from down under because it definitely proved to be the right direction.

Remote support ...

Starting from where the sun rose first in our circle of supporters, our friends in Australia, going on to Singapore followed by India – Achala. What could I say when she found ways to connect on Face Time/Skype despite the 18 hours' time difference and seeing patients, cried when I cried and laughed her heartwarming laugh irrespective of what people thought in her clinic.

Mary Jane, the regular messages from her always brought a smile and her Aussie trooper did us all proud. She developed a huge fan following amongst all the regular contributors in the blog as she gave words to everyone's thoughts despite being a stranger.

Marion made beautiful connection by using German translate when she couldn't understand something and then coming back to me with her understanding that was truly touching.

Cirsten, now in Hamburg, stayed connected with regular support, even sponsoring Lavanya's fund raising efforts all the way from there.

Jayshree – her patience with my endless talking, texting helped us through some of the most difficult phases. She has this amazing ability to listen quietly, providing lasting comfort.

Shilpi's regular messages, mails, FB chats were huge boosters as we felt her feeling our pains and rejoicing in our joy. Shilpi and Jayshree, unknown to me, connected with each other and touched us all by arriving in Kolkata for just one day to spend entirely with me when I lost my sister. Yes, two perfect strangers realized they were both in Singapore, got in touch with each other and decided they needed to be with me in my moment of tremendous loss.

Krishna, Jayshree's husband – we will remain forever grateful to him for the Tirupati walk and one on one with Balaji for Lavanya's health. Alka and Shilpi have had this

271

prayer chain and chanting on and I have no clue as to who the people involved were and where they were, but we stay grateful to all those unknown people.

Rachna, gave up something so precious that we used to share, that coffee, until our girl recovered. I told her to treat herself to a huge mug.

Usha's messages every morning and evening with clockwork precision whatever else was going on in her life, warmed us with the knowledge that she was with us all the way. She knew the chemo schedule, drugs involved and side effects as well as we did.

Joel and my brother-in-law, Hemadri deserve awards for keeping a sick teen entertained by just talking to her whenever she felt 'bored' in the hospital and sometimes even at home, keeping all that they were doing on hold. It both amused and touched me when sitting between both our kids, each glued to their respective phones, an exasperated me complained at the unfairness of the situation, only to hear a reply, "Shhh don't disturb, it's Joel uncle's turn at 'words with friends'." Joel managed to keep not one but two kids occupied by building words across continents, giving us time to catch our breath.

Deepak's regular mails to Varun and me were heartwarming as were Karthik's calls. They brought back memories from the time they stood by us during our first experience with leukemia in Mumbai.

Poulomi, Mamta and Angelika showed amazing heart when they donated to the charities Lavanya had been supporting through the years in her honor.

Aditi, Simran and Isha, the three teens from Mumbai who despite their studies, homework and tests connected whenever they could. It was fun to hear Lavanya giggling either early mornings or late nights, with the twelve hour plus time difference. I appreciated Radhika's wise words and FB prayer chain that generated endless prayers.

When all roads led to Cupertino ...

Our friends whether visiting anywhere in America made it a point to make that little detour to head to Cupertino or Stanford. Mind it, the United States is a vast country but distance didn't bother them. Alka from Singapore, Swarnali, Shrey, Rajesh, Joel, Karthik, Prema, Snegha, Meenakshi, Aparna from Mumbai, Saurabh, Surbhi and Macarena from Melbourne, Gaurav from Minnesota, Nafis from New Jersey – they took time out of their busy schedules, multiple appointments to spend time with us. United States Postal Services, Fedex and others received good business when our friends from across the world sent presents and cards and Lavanya realized that a sick child received more gifts than a birthday child.

Kate, our social worker in the hospital gives social work a new meaning, with her prompt replies to all our queries, a personal touch here and a little word there she made the entire treatment much easier. Stanford Children's Hospital, Dr Lacayo, Dr Dahl, Dr Mahapatra, the nurse practitioners and nurses, Carly, Daisy, Angela, Cam, Marianne, Sheila, Sara, Jen, Sadie, Jonah and the staff in One North, day hospital, PICU, appointment setters, the trio of the lovely receptionists in the Bass Center, the valet parking boys, the boom gate security had all become a huge part of our lives in our quest to cure. I would always stay grateful to Dr Lacayo for managing Lavanya's therapy beautifully so she had a life beyond leukemia and its treatment. She visited her dream destination France with her teacher and French class for two weeks and gained a French family there who hosted her. We were greatly appreciative of her French Teacher Sarah Finck who bravely took on the responsibility of letting a child undergoing therapy join the trip and make concessions when she couldn't walk as much as the others or needed to rest between tours due to her condition of avascular necrosis.

The friends who regularly lifted our spirits with warm beautiful words of love, encouragement and support – Priya Devotta, Priya Desai, Rupa, Aparna, Shilpi, Alka, Achala, Lisa, Christine, Mary Jane, Usha, Jayshree, Radhika. No words could thank them enough. Those who had been silent on the website, but we knew that they had been with us; we extended our grateful thanks to them, too. We have been touched by love and blessings both expressed regularly and unexpressed, but evident.

We began maintenance in January 2014 lasting 18 months, entailing daily oral chemo, once a week intra muscular chemo shot, once a month IV infusion and once in three months lumbar puncture. It was not easy, but it was easier than the past intense treatment of weekly lumbar punctures, 72 hour long infusions involving frequent transfusions and blood draw. Eventually Lavanya had to give up all physical activities like running, basketball and any other sport that she might have played due to her bone condition. Our 17 year old adjusted to chronic pain due to dead bones with a quiet acceptance, "At least I am not in the hospital all the time."

Lavanya was accepted in multiple renowned colleges across America starting with UC Berkeley in the west coast to Georgetown in the east. She chose to head to Georgetown in the fall of 2015 to study in the Edmund Walsh School of Foreign Services and delightedly prepared to begin her life cancer free, the only reminder being the monthly checkup which will taper off to once a year eventually to carry on for the next ten years or until she is 25. She would rather forget the associated issues that have come with the disease and treatment, to lead as much of a normal life as possible. She dreams big and we are happy to add fuel to them and our dear circle joins us to applaud and celebrate her.

I have learnt much from everyone, starting with my girl, my boy, my hubby to each one of our friends, family and our children's teachers and staff. I learnt about the goodness of humanity, the greatness of hearts, the power of prayers, the magic of positivity, the truth of belief and the marvel of medical science. I thanked God for proving time and again that when he brings you to it, he sees you through it – you just have to accept all his presents with love.

Epilogue

"You don't reach points in life at which everything is sorted out for us. I believe in endings that should suggest our stories always continue."

Lauren Oliver

In August 2015, a few weeks prior to departure for college the port was surgically removed and the one last connection to chemotherapy detached forever. I watched as Lavanya answered the pre-op questions to the nurses and then the anesthetists to follow it up with a request of her own, "May I push my own anesthesia under your supervision?" The anesthetists looked amused and asked, "Why and do you often do that?" On hearing Lavanya's reply of the taste of anesthesia due the port proximity to throat as well as general wellbeing associated with her own administration as against the anesthetist's, the doctors realized that it was safe in their presence and close supervision and hence agreed. They laughed amongst themselves, "Oh she is eyeing our jobs!" Lavanya was told to get on the bed so that she could be pushed to OR from pre-op and our girl said, "But why? I am fine, I can walk. Can I walk?" This initiated few calls to supervisors, head nurse, floor in charge with whispers of, "Patient wants to walk. The patient wants to walk! Huh!" Standing next to them I could almost hear the head nurse's response on the phone, "What? Patient wants to walk?"

So we waited for the head nurse to come to review the patient and when she saw her healthy young patient standing tall on her two steady feet ready to waltz all the way to the OR she murmured, "Oh well, our patients in pediatric surgery are in no state to walk to OR, but you look good, so I will help you." Saying so the lovely, elderly petite head nurse who barely reached my daughter's shoulder held her around her waist with her dainty arms and walked her to the OR followed by pre-op nurse, OR nurse, floor nurse, chief anesthetist, assistant anesthetist, a nurse pushing the empty bed alongside and yours truly.

I bid them adieu at the fork of the corridor and walked into the waiting room with its big black board giving surgery status with green blinking lights and I was back to the feel of an airport terminal and when the port was placed more than two years ago. Only now I wore a smile, sipping my hot latte, warmed by the thoughtful, expert patient care and cherishing the sight of that last grin I saw on our girl's face before she and her entourage disappeared behind the closed doors of the OR.